This book is dedicated to the innovative employers who have helped refine a better way to meet the health needs of their employees by using high quality and cost effective methods. They have helped make the 20/20 LifeStyles Wellness Program what it is today.

# TABLE OF CONTENTS

# LOWERING CORPORATE HEALTH CARE CO$T

How to successfully reverse
the ever increasing costs of
corporate health care.

Mark Dedomenico, MD
Barry Wolborsky, PhD

Published by PRO Sports Club, Bellevue and Seattle, Washington.
In association with Better Life Press, Seattle Washington.

proclub.com
2020LifeStyles.com

ISBN: Hardback: 978-0-9909514-6-9

Metadata: 1 Health/fitness. 2 Diet/exercise/nutrition. 3 Metabolic disease, high cholesterol, hypertension, heart disease, diabetes. 4 Weight loss/weight management. 5 Reversing metabolic disease/natural permanent weight loss. 6 Mark Dedomenico, MD, cardiovascular surgeon, researcher, author. 7 Barry Wolborsky, PhD, psychologist, addictions expert, author.

Cover design: Molly Owen
Interior layout design: Molly Owen

# CHAPTER 6: THE 20/20 LIFESTYLES WELLNESS PROGRAM

# CHAPTER 7: ELEMENTS OF THE 20/20 LIFESTYLES PROGRAM

# CHAPTER 8: 20/20 LIFESTYLES PREVENTION MODULES

# CHAPTER 9: 20/20 LIFESTYLES TREATMENT MODULES-PART 1

# CHAPTER 10: 20/20 LIFESTYLES TREATMENT MODULES-PART 2

# CHAPTER 11: 20/20 LIFESTYLES TREATMENT MODULES-PART 3

# CHAPTER 12: 20/20 LIFESTYLES TREATMENT MODULES-PART 4

# CHAPTER 13: A REAL-LIFE CASE STUDY

# APPENDIX A

# APPENDIX B

# APPENDIX C

# ACKNOWLEDGEMENTS

The authors wish to thank Robert Davenport, Wellness Consultant for Wells Fargo employee benefits, for his input and guidance throughout the process.

We would also like to thank our panel of local CFOs and CEOs who gave us input on the current state of healthcare cost management and wellness programs in a wide variety of companies.

We are also grateful to Judy Crane and Jen Masterson for keeping us on track and dealing with the mega re-writes that finally created this book.

Additionally to our panel of professionals who carefully read the manuscript and helped us simplify and clarify the topics in this book; thank you.

Lastly we would like acknowledge the staff of the 20/20 LifeStyles Program, the Counseling Center at PRO Sports Club and all the dietitians, counselors, physicians and exercise physiologists at PRO Sports Club who carefully read this book and gave us the feedback we needed to correct errors and include the important details we had omitted. Thank you all!

# INTRODUCTION TO HEALTH

If you want to really cut your company's healthcare costs, then I invite you to read this book. This book is not about "pie in the sky" approaches to reducing your company's medical expenses; it is about tried and proven methods that actually work and how implementing those methods will have a positive impact on your bottom line.

As a doctor and a businessman, I was motivated to find answers--to develop a wellness program that made a difference. The doctor in me set out to find ways of reducing needless illnesses that employees endured due to ignorance or poor medical advice, and the businessman in me realized that improving employee health would lead to a significant return on investment (ROI) for companies everywhere.

Like other business men and women, I was alarmed at the rapid increase in medical costs. But as a doctor I could see that if companies were wise enough to change the way they addressed healthcare, they would become more productive and profitable, and the resulting domino effect could eventually have benefits on all companies, and eventually, on our nation's economy.

I know that in the past you've often heard companies and individuals claim that they had solutions to your healthcare cost problems. You've probably even tried some of those "solutions."But I'll bet the result has largely been the same; that your healthcare costs continued to rise year after year. Right? Well, if I'm on the money or even close on this topic so far, I'm going to ask that you suspend your skepticism for just a few minutes and read on.

First, a bit of background: When I began my career as a cardiovascular surgeon, I saw the disastrous results of metabolic disease. I worked with patients on a daily basis who had heart disease, strokes, and diabetes. I also knew that this pain and suffering was self-caused by unhealthy lifestyles and that if those lifestyles were changed, the diseases would be prevented or cured. But the devil was in the details; I found that lifestyles were extremely resistant to change.

After years of seeing this parade of misery and illness in my practice, I became more and more interested in preventing these diseases, rather than just treating them. It was then that I started meeting with a very talented group of doctors, psychologists, dietitians, and exercise physiologists to discuss a plan to prevent and even cure metabolic disease. The result of those meetings became what we now call the 20/20 LifeStyles Program. As of this writing, 20/20 LifeStyles has continued for well over 20 years and has cured metabolic disease in more than 10,000 individuals. Without the 20/20 LifeStyles Program, most of these people would have wound up being treated by a cardiovascular surgeon or some other specialist. They would have had multiple surgeries, procedures, tests, and hospitalizations. Their healthcare costs would have been astronomical and their lives miserable.

Having developed and refined the techniques to make the 20/20 LifeStyles Program so successful, our talented team launched the 20/20 LifeStyles Wellness Program. This program's success is based on what we have learned over the last two decades while working with people who are just like your employees (in fact, they may have been some of your employees).

If you currently have a wellness program, it's probably structured in a way that it attempts to prevent employees from developing various diseases. The problem, however, is that 80% of your healthcare dollars are spent on the 20% of your employees and insured families who already have those chronic diseases. These individuals are a constant drag on your healthcare expenses. But the good news is this: 20/20 LifeStyles has a proven record of curing many of these chronic diseases.

The keys to our success are motivation, competence, and trust. No wellness program can be successful in your company without motivating your employees and insured family members to participate. Poor participation in wellness programs virtually guarantees their failure. Dealing with medical issues can be extremely confusing. Your employees need competent professionals to lead them through the lack of information, conflicting claims, and the frustration of dealing with the healthcare system. Trust is only achieved when your employees or family members know that their wellness professional is not only competent, but actually cares about them.

This book contains an overview of the state of healthcare economics as they exist today, and it also features stories gathered from companies and individual employees of companies that have had experience with the 20/20 LifeStyles Wellness Program. It describes our techniques and treatment modules.

In most chapters you will find two basic sections:

1. A personal account by an employee from various businesses that reflects some of the issues in healthcare today.

2. A fact-finding section that reveals relevant healthcare data, medical facts, and statistics, as well as new methodologies in wellness and new approaches to contain healthcare expenses.

Chapter One details the dismal history of the attempts to control healthcare costs. This chapter lists facts and figures that might be a bit difficult to read, but we feel it's important for you to review what has been tried and why it failed. Without that information it could be difficult for you to understand what is needed to really make a change.

Chapters Two through Seven describe the elements of a wellness program that are necessary in dealing with the various healthcare problems experienced in your company.

Chapter Eight explains the 20/20 LifeStyles Wellness Program Illness and Injury Prevention Program.

Chapters Nine through Twelve cover the 20/20 LifeStyles Wellness Program Treatment Modules. These modules are carefully designed to treat your employees' specific medical conditions. We show you how this can be done effectively and in a cost-efficient manner, and we always give you ROI data on treatment modules.

Chapter Thirteen presents the actual results for a company using the 20/20 LifeStyles Wellness Program, and the results are dramatic.

In summary, I wrote this book because I feel that we've developed a working solution to the problem of runaway healthcare costs. I hope that in these pages you'll be able to find some real-world answers that help you improve your company's wellness program, improve your employees' health, and control your medical costs.

# CHAPTER 1

## WE SELL IDEAS

---

### OUR ANNUAL COMPANY REPORT
#### *Daniel - Executive Assistant to the CFO of a Local Software Company*

I work for a software company that has 427 employees. A few months ago I was promoted to executive assistant for our CFO. Our annual meeting was coming up soon and I was helping my boss prepare our annual financial report.

I kept re-reading our annual report, hoping I'd find that I made a mistake in preparing it. Our company was doing well and business was good; we even had a backlog of work. The supply of skilled technical labor was above normal, and our wages were up only 1.5% year-over-year. We were able to raise our average hourly contract rate by 3% due to greater efficiency, mostly related to better employees. It was hard for me to believe that our year-over-year profit was down 1.7%. I thought I had done something wrong in my calculations.

I knew I had only a week before I presented the report to my CFO and just 10 days before our annual company meeting. I also knew that when I presented those results, I'd better have some answers. I started to drill into the numbers and found that total employee costs were up 3.35%. And yet salaries and hiring costs were up only 1.5%, which was less than half of the total increase.

Drilling down further into the numbers, I found that our employee health care costs were up 8%, our worker's compensation costs were up 11%, and to my amazement, our long-term and short-term disability costs had risen 12%.

Being a medically self-insured company, these costs directly affected our bottom line. To make matters worse, our unemployment insurance costs had increased, and our absenteeism rate was up as well. To get some answers, I quickly set up a meeting with our insurance provider and our HR director.

After that meeting, it became clear to me that healthcare costs were slowly but surely eating away at our bottom line. Unless we found a solution to this problem it would continue to decrease our profits year-after-year.

Our HR director explained to me that in 2008, when it was easy to hire good employees, we had established a medical cost-sharing plan with our employees. Under that plan employees had to contribute to both healthcare insurance costs and medical visit costs. Since that time, we had been unable to increase the employee share of health insurance cost because to get the best people in our field we had to offer benefits competitive to what larger companies offered. As I mentioned before, our business model only succeeds if we hire the best.

Our HR director and insurer also told me that five years ago they had established a wellness program to control healthcare costs. We offered our employees a $200 annual discount on their share of health insurance costs to participate. To be eligible, they had to fill out an online health risk assessment questionnaire and have a screening. The screening consisted of having a technician measure their biometrics to determine the employee's body weight, height, blood pressure, and draw blood to determine their blood glucose and cholesterol levels. If health problems were discovered during this process, the employee would see his or her personal physician for treatment, and a wellness program person then monitored the employee by phone.

I asked if we had tracked the results of that program over the five years since we established it. They replied that was difficult to do since healthcare costs had been rising every year. However they believed that our healthcare costs would have increased faster without the wellness program.

The cost of the wellness program was $45 per employee per month or $540 a year. When you add the $200 health insurance discount that was $740 per employee per year. A cost to my company of over $230,000. What bothered me most was that there was no way to really determine whether or not the program was controlling our costs and there was certainly no way to determine if we were getting a positive ROI on this annual expense.

I also found out that only 46% of our employees participated in the wellness program. There was really no way to tell if that 46% was mostly healthy individuals who just wanted the $200 annual discount or if it was actually helping the less healthy employees that were spending the majority of our healthcare dollars.

At this point it became very obvious to me that my boss needed to get involved in managing my company's healthcare.

After I researched our healthcare costs, I began to investigate possible solutions for controlling those ever-increasing costs. And when I met with my boss I was prepared. I had developed a plan that I thought would get control of those costs. I told my CFO that our HR director and I had investigated a number of wellness programs and we were most impressed by the 20/20 LifeStyles Wellness Program. The program's results were quite impressive; they had successfully treated over 10,000 individuals with metabolic disorders. And best of all, it actually showed a positive return on investment. None of the other programs that we had researched demonstrated anything like these results. My CEO was very enthusiastic about my report and asked that I set up a meeting with 20/20 LifeStyles.

During that meeting, 20/20 LifeStyles told us the first step would be to meet with all of our management team in order to find out their most pressing concerns about employee healthcare. They told us that these concerns were often related to absenteeism and presenteeism[1] and that for the program to succeed, it was vital that 20/20 LifeStyles have full management support of the program. Next they would conduct a number of focus groups for employees and their insured family members to discover their likes and dislikes of the previous wellness program. They felt it was important to meet with those who had participated in our previous program but even more important to meet with those employees who had not participated. This would help them determine if we were mainly spending our wellness dollars on the well, while the less healthy employees avoided the program. At that point they would meet with us to propose a program specifically designed for our company.

After hearing the plan, my CFO gave our HR director the green light and told me to keep him informed as we progressed.

Well, we've been running the 20/20 LifeStyles Wellness Program for a little over a year now, and we just finished meeting with our healthcare insurer. All I can say is WOW! Our medical costs are down 11% as opposed to last year's increase of 8%. Our workmen's compensation cost and absenteeism are both also down over 10% as opposed to last year's 11% increase, and our disability costs are now stable. Our productivity is up 6% (based on hours spent per dollars earned), our staff turnover rate is down 4.5%, and the 20/20 LifeStyles Wellness Program was rated excellent by 82% of our participating

---

1. There are numerous definitions of presenteeism, but they all center on the concept of the employee being at work while impaired. See Chapter Two on "The Hidden Costs" for a more detailed explanation.

employees. My boss can't wait to present the final results to our CEO.

---

The following pages require some explanation. They consist of facts and figures related to attempts made by government, industry, think tanks, and others to control healthcare costs. Reading this section of the book will give you an understanding of just how many promising ideas about healthcare have failed. That way the next time someone approaches you with their "good idea" to reduce healthcare costs, you can say, "That has been tried, it didn't work."

# INCREASING HEALTHCARE COSTS-- DECREASING PROFITS

Healthcare costs will increase 6.8% in 2015[2]. This is due to several factors, including the improving U.S. economy, the increasing cost of hospitalizations, the increasing cost of emergency room and urgent care visits, the development of new extremely high-priced specialty drugs, physicians becoming part of hospital networks (which increases the cost of physician visits), and the cost of medical information technology problems.

The U. S. economy is recovering from a severe recession with high levels of unemployment, but the unemployment rate is expected to settle at about 4.8%[3]. The improvement in employment has allowed many individuals who had deferred medical treatment to obtain it. Increased medical costs, however, lag behind the unemployment rate recovery by about four-to-five years, so we are just beginning to see the increases[4]. Based on this lag and the initiation of the Affordable Care Act, we can

---

2. *PricewaterhouseCooper's Health Research Institute, June 24, 2014.*
3. *Federal Reserve Board, September 2015.*
4. *PricewaterhouseCooper's Health Research Institute, June 24, 2014.*

expect larger than normal healthcare cost increases for the next 4 to 5 years.

Drug manufacturers have developed specialty drugs that are extremely costly. Amazingly, because of government requirements, it costs about two billion dollars to bring a new drug to market. Consequently drug manufacturers must price that development cost into the cost of the drug, based on the term of the patent and the life expectancy of the product. Some examples of these drugs are Sanofi's Zaltrap for colon cancer[5], which costs $132,000 per year, for life; Gilead's Sovaldi for hepatitis[6], which costs $84,000 for a 12-week treatment regimen; Teva's Copazone for multiple sclerosis[7], which costs $72,000 per year for life; and Alexion's Soliris for an immune system disorder, which costs over $400,000 per year for life. Add to this the cost of physician visits and testing to administer and monitor these drugs, plus the treatments and hospitalizations required to deal with the side effects of these drugs, and the cost becomes staggering. It is obvious that for a small or medium-sized company just one employee using one of these drugs can have a major impact on the bottom line, year after year. Unfortunately this trend will continue into the foreseeable future. Frightening, isn't it?

Insurers and government entities have continually squeezed medical providers over and over. As a result these providers are examining options to increase or at least stabilize their profitability. Many doctors who have been in private practice find that becoming employed by hospitals actually increases their income. Hospital-employed doctors then refer patients to their hospital for all testing, imaging, and services (such as physical therapy or rehabilitation). Hospitals find that by buying out medical practices, especially primary

5. Colon cancer affects 1 person in 20, and overweight individuals have a significantly increased risk for colon cancer.
6. Hepatitis affects 1 person in 100 (3,000,000 adults).
7. Multiple sclerosis affects 1.25 in 1000, and lifetime cost of treatment is $1.2 million.

care practices, they can dramatically increase their referral rates for high-cost medical procedures, tests, and surgeries. The cost of these hospital-based services can run up to 400% higher than the same service obtained through an independent provider[8]. Even without tests or hospital services, treatment costs billed by hospital employed providers range from 30% higher to over 100% higher[9].

In 2009, as part of the President's "overhaul" of U. S. healthcare, electronic healthcare records were mandated. A study by the Wharton School at the University of Pennsylvania concluded that current technology could increase costs without improving care[10], and this cost increase is occurring. In 2011, the cost of installing an electronic health records system ranged from $33,000 to $70,000 per provider plus annual maintenance costs of about $17,000 per year[11], and these costs have continued to increase. Additional expenses not considered are the time lost by healthcare professionals learning the new and updated systems and maintaining them.

Furthermore there are major problems with healthcare information technology systems as they now exist, which will need to be addressed at some point and will be very costly. These include lack of compatibility of systems, data security concerns, and lack of usability by physicians. Additionally the theft of computer data from under-protected medical databases means you could be paying for medical care delivered to a fraudulent non-employee who has used stolen healthcare information to obtain treatment. Neither you nor your employee would be aware of this theft.

This list is certainly not all-inclusive. We haven't mentioned

---

8. *A hospital-based MRI imaging study will cost about $4,000. The same service from an independent provider was $900.*
9. *National Institute for Health Care Reform, Research Brief no.16 June 2014.*
10. *Wharton School, University of Pennsylvania, June 2009.*
11. *Niel S. Fleming, et. al., "The Financial and Non-Financial Costs..." Health Affairs, March 2011.*

the promotion of off-label use of drugs, the cost of high tech medical equipment, the increased cost of complex medical procedures, or the increased use of expensive medical testing. It is quite clear that these expenses will continue to rise and your costs will continue to increase. If you feel these out-of-control costs are startling, keep reading.

The current cost of healthcare in the U. S. is equivalent to between 18% and 20% of our current Gross Domestic Product (GDP). The next two highest industrialized countries are France and Germany, which are at about 12% of their GDP[12]. Additionally, the growth of the U.S. healthcare costs is predicted to be between 1.2% and 2.4% greater than the national growth of our GDP[13], and this is expected to continue for the foreseeable future. That means that unless healthcare costs are contained, they will equal the total U.S. GDP between 2047 and 2081--or to put it another way--every dollar you generate will go toward healthcare!

The Affordable Care Act of 2010 has caused business healthcare costs to increase 5% to 15%[14]. Even at current levels, ACA will cost $675 billion over the next 10 years, which will almost certainly require new tax increases. Keep in mind, it is impossible to predict future costs of the ACA since it will undoubtedly be modified many times, and it is likely that current estimates are very low. This, of course, makes planning for future healthcare costs even more difficult.

And if that weren't bad enough, as part of the ACA, a very large number of tests and procedures have been added to the list of "preventive health services." These are medical expenses that must be paid in full by all health insurance plans without co-pays or deductibles. This list consists of 15 procedures for all adults, an additional 22 procedures for

12. *World Bank Total Health Expenditures.*
13. *A. Chandra, J. Holmes, J. Skinner, "Is This Time Different? The Slowdown in Healthcare Spending," presented at The Brookings Institute 2013 fall conference.*
14. *International Foundation of Employee Benefit Plans, 2013*

women, and 26 procedures for children. See appendix A for a complete list of these procedures and their itemized costs.

As we mentioned previously, hospital-owned medical services cost about double the cost of the same services provided at an independent provider's office. For a breakdown of these costs, see appendix B.

Since there are no deductibles or co-pays for these procedures, 100% of their cost will be paid for by your company. As you can see, this will cause an immediate and permanent increase in your healthcare costs. In Chapter Eight, the chapter on prevention, we will discuss how by contracting with individual providers, you can greatly minimize these costs.

Individuals in government and business and many insurers have recognized the problem of out-of-control healthcare costs and have attempted to mitigate or solve it. Many different approaches have been tried, but healthcare costs still increase.

# ATTEMPTS AT CONTROLLING HEALTHCARE COSTS

In this section we will discuss the major attempts at managing healthcare costs in the last 50 years. This is, by necessity, only a partial list. A complete listing could fill many books. While some of these attempts may seem interesting and innovative, others might strike you as unreasonable or even ridiculous. But they all have one thing in common: they attempt to control the costs of treating illness and disease, rather than preventing or curing it.

In 1971 President Nixon imposed price and wage controls on the entire economy with special mechanisms designed to contain healthcare costs. Nixon also proposed a Comprehensive Health Insurance Plan that was given serious consideration by Congress but was later dropped after Nixon's untimely departure from office. In 1975 the healthcare cost controls were lifted after a pledge was made by the healthcare industry to control costs voluntarily[15]. We know how well that worked!

In 1977 President Carter proposed hospital cost containment. In 1979, he introduced a plan that included minimum standards for benefits and established mandatory employer contributions, a new Federal Healthcare program to replace Medicaid and Medicare and cover the elderly, the disabled, and all low-income individuals. This was in response to the rapid increase in healthcare costs after Nixon's controls were lifted. That legislation was defeated by the healthcare industry's promising once again to voluntarily control costs. Amazing, isn't it?

In 1993 the Federal Government tried again to regulate healthcare costs. President Clinton introduced the Health Security Act, which mandated that employers pay 80% of premiums (up to a maximum cost of 7.9% of total payroll). The family share of premiums was not to exceed 3.9% of income. The plan was to be financed by substantial Medicare and Medicaid savings, an increase in tobacco taxes, and cross-subsidies among employers within risk pools. The plan was defeated in Congress due to its negative effects on small business[16]. Medicare and Medicaid savings? Really? Were they serious?

In 2010, President Obama was able to pass the Affordable Care Act. Although there are many conflicting estimates of increased healthcare costs due to the ACA, those estimates all remain very questionable. Premiums will only be held to current levels of increase because the insurance providers have access to Federal funds until 2017. After that, premiums will rise much faster! Some estimates say premiums may double and at this point the number of uninsured Americans could

15. K. Davis, G. Anderson, D. Rowland, and E. Steinberg, *Health Care Cost Containment* (Baltimore: The Johns Hopkins University Press, 1990).
16. Congressional Research Service, *Health Care Reform: President Clinton's Health Security Act*, (Washington, D. C.: Congressional Research Service, 1993).

again rise dramatically due to the unaffordable premiums. Unbelievable isn't it? So much for government efforts.

In the late 1980s, insurers introduced Health Maintenance Organizations (HMOs) and Preferred Provider Organizations (PPOs). These were designed to control costs by impaneling providers, who would then accept lower reimbursement schedules in order to treat patients belonging to the HMO or PPO. Many plans also required authorization and monitoring by the insurer's medical departments before patients could see specialists or obtain costly tests, procedures, and surgeries (managed care). These measures temporarily moderated the rate of healthcare cost increases but were strongly disliked by patients, who felt that their doctors and not their insurers should be making decisions about their medical care.

In the mid-1990s, with unemployment at a very low level and companies competing for employees, these programs were modified to make them more palatable to employees. However, it should be noted that currently almost all insurance is still delivered through providers who participate in insurer networks. Currently less than 1% of employees and their families are covered under plans that do not use a provider network. Since almost all medical treatment is provided by in-network providers, we wonder how this actually cuts costs.

Integrated Managed Healthcare Consortiums are fully contained managed health organizations such as Group Health Cooperative or Kaiser Permanente. They own hospitals and employ healthcare providers. The first of this type of organization was started in Los Angeles in 1908 to insure workers on the California aqueduct system. Many of these organizations continue to provide healthcare services and have found a place in the overall healthcare system. Data is sparse on any employer savings due to the use of these types of healthcare systems.

Many insurance plans offer case management services for patients with chronic illnesses like diabetes, high blood pressure, and heart disease. These plans attempt to direct the patient to receive timely and effective medical care for their illness so that hospitalizations and emergency room visits are decreased. There is little consensus regarding the ability of these programs to control costs[17]. In other words, they are not effective.

Additionally most companies have raised deductibles and co-pay levels for their health insurance plans in an attempt to control their ever-increasing healthcare costs. A deductible is the amount of money the insured must spend on eligible healthcare expenses before the insurance plan begins to pay. Co-pays are either fixed amounts or percentages of the cost of each healthcare expense that the insured has to pay. In 2014 over 60% of employers were currently either offering or considering offering only high deductible plans[18] (plans with deductibles over $2,000 per year).

High performance (high value) provider networks rely on data that measures provider performance[19]. They attempt to identify providers who deliver high quality and cost-effective healthcare. Plans vary in their use of high-performance networks. Some plans have tiers of payment, based on whether or not a provider is included in their standard network, their high- performance network, or is not in their network. Other plans will only cover medical services provided by their high-performance providers. In selecting a high-performance provider network, an employee's cost for his health insurance premiums would be lower, but he would have to use a more limited network of providers and facilities. Estimates of healthcare cost savings using high-performance provider networks range from 0% to 20%. That range of savings, from

17. *Comparative Effectiveness of Case Management for Adults With Medical Illness and Complex Care Needs, 2011, Agency for Healthcare Research and Quality, U. S. Dept. Health and Human Services.*
18. *PwC 2014 Health and Well-Being Touchstone Survey.*
19. *Attempts to systematically measure provider performance are extremely arbitrary. Often different measurement systems produce very different results.*

almost no savings 20%, makes you wonder about the real value of these plans.

We agree with the concept that the most effective healthcare will result in the least expensive healthcare. There is no doubt that some providers and institutions have much lower complications and hospital re-admissions rates than others. There are two problems we have seen in these attempts, and perhaps they are the reason for the 0% to 20% range. The first is the difficulty of actually identifying the best providers and institutions, and the second is the tendency to choose the least-expensive provider in order to save money. High-performance provider networks are a good idea, but the devil is in the details.

Consumer-driven health plans operate on the theory that making the insured more aware of healthcare choices and costs will help limit those costs. The consumer-driven plan does this by having the employee involved in the payment of healthcare costs. This is accomplished by having a healthcare insurance plan with a very high deductible, which is partially compensated with a company-funded medical savings account (MSA) or healthcare savings account (HSA). Initial payments on any benefit-year would come out of the MSA or HSA, which contains employer plus employee funds. It is believed that the employees will take a greater interest in limiting their healthcare costs because they are spending their own money.

There are a number of reasons why consumer-driven health plans have not been successful at controlling healthcare costs. First, if you offer plan options, this type of plan attracts the healthier employees, while those with medical problems opt for more traditional plans. This tends to drive up the cost of the traditional plans[20]. Since 80% of healthcare dollars are spent on 20% of your employees, this plan might actually lead to cost increases rather than decreases. Second, this plan assumes that the least expensive medical care is the best medical care, which is

20. *Pepperdine University, Graziadio Business Review, Volume 7, issue 3.*

not usually the case. Missed diagnoses, false positives, treatment side effects, and ineffective treatment rapidly raise medical costs. Third, most employees don't have the knowledge to make good medical choices without guidance. The medical field is complex, and treatment recommendations vary greatly. Relying on the internet for medical guidance rarely produces a good outcome. Last, since there is almost no way to know medical costs in advance, the employee can't choose providers based on costs. Recently an employee at a company we work with had to undergo two identical medical procedures a month apart. The procedures were performed by the same doctor in the same facility using the same equipment. We noticed that the two charges differed by $800. We called the providers billing department to discuss this but were told that there may have been complications or that additional equipment had to be used. When we told them that the procedures were identical and asked them to itemize everything that was done, they agreed to remove the $800 mistaken charge. We have a major problem with the fact that medical costs are so difficult to obtain from providers.

Eighty-eight percent (88%) of all employers either have or are planning to implement a wellness program. Average employee participation in these plans was 54% to 57%. Ninety percent (90%) of these employers do not have sufficient data or do not measure their return on investment (ROI) for their wellness programs[21]. Based on this lack of data, the value of these plans is highly questionable.

Additionally 53% offer disease management programs; the most common are diabetes, chronic obstructive pulmonary disease and cardiac. Most employers consider their diabetes program as the most valuable disease-management program. Eighty-seven percent (87%) of employers do not have sufficient data or do not measure their return on investment (ROI) for their disease-management programs. Once again,

21. PwC 2014 Health and Well-Being Touchstone Survey.

we wonder if these programs reduce costs or increase costs.

The list of healthcare cost "solutions" above is quite impressive. Government entities, insurers, employers, universities, and independent think tanks have all contributed to these "solutions." However, even with all those attempted solutions, the bottom line is that healthcare costs are predicted to grow by 6.8% in 2015 and these "solutions" are not working.

# CHAPTER 2

## I'M HERE BUT NOT ALL THERE

### I WAS THE BEST

*Tony - V. P. Marketing for a Snack Food Company*

I remember it was a Thursday afternoon and the stack of unfinished work on my desk was huge. I felt overwhelmed with unfinished work and afraid to look at my unanswered emails. I was 52 years old and the vice-president of marketing for a regional snack food manufacturer, but I felt like I was 80.

The snack food business is very competitive, but I always used to stay one step ahead of the competition. I also used to be the company go-to man, not only for marketing problems but problems in any area of the company. I was good at analyzing a situation and suggesting solutions that nobody else had thought of. Then things began to change. Over the last few years, my co-workers stopped asking for my input. I had been the main driver of sales in this company, but now, I wasn't doing a good job of it. I felt down, and our sales were down. Over the last few years I had somehow slowed down more and more. I was tired from morning to night, and just walking from my parking place to the office left me out of breath.

I had played football in high school and had stayed fairly athletic. I played racquetball a couple of times a week and golf on weekends. I'd been pretty healthy all my life. I never even got a cold. I thought I was "bullet proof." But then, responsibilities at work and a 40-pound weight gain put an end to all that. I ate and drank what I wanted, when I wanted, and just didn't have the time or energy for exercise anymore.

About four years ago, I got the first cold that I had in over 10 years, and it was really bad. My temperature spiked at 102, my body ached all over, I couldn't stop coughing, and I couldn't sleep. After about three days of that, my wife insisted that I go to the doctor. She wouldn't let me out of it. She even made the appointment and drove me there. The doctor examined me, took some blood, prescribed an antibiotic, and told me to come back in a week.

Well, a week later, I was feeling better and thought I would cancel my appointment, but my illness had really scared my wife. She insisted I go, in fact she came with me. The doctor told me the reason that my cold was so severe was that my blood sugar was high and that the bacteria in my body thrived in a high sugar environment. He said I was diabetic and also told me I had high blood pressure, high cholesterol, and was 45 pounds overweight.

I was stunned. My dad had diabetes, which caused him to have several of his toes amputated and kidney failure. He died of a stroke at the age of 60. I thought, My God, I'm 52 years old, that only gives me eight more years.

The doctor said I needed to go on medication for my high blood pressure, diabetes, and high cholesterol. The only pills that I had ever taken were a couple of Tylenols in the morning after a long, hard-drinking sales dinner. He also advised me to lose weight. He gave me the prescriptions and told me to make another appointment with him in 60 days.

Before I left, the doctor warned me that the medications had side effects, which might be uncomfortable, but he also said that if I didn't take them, I could wind up disabled or dead. But I hated them.

The blood pressure pills caused my feet to swell and hurt. One of the medications constantly upset my stomach, and I never really felt good.

Being a busy guy, it took me about four months to get back to see the doctor. My blood pressure was down to 140 over 90 and my weight was down five pounds. He told me he'd call me back with the results of my blood tests. When he called about a week later and told me my cholesterol was down to 210 and my blood sugar was 120. The doctor said we had made some progress and he'd see me in six months.

Well, you know me, six months became a year, and I had to see him because my prescriptions had expired and my wife kept asking when I was going back to see the doctor.

After that, I'd see him about once a year, mainly because my wife would "remind" me. Over time I managed to gain back the five pounds I lost plus another 10. Then, my doctor had to add another medication to control my blood pressure and now I had to inject myself with insulin, which I really hated.

In all honesty, I wasn't very good at taking my pills or injecting the insulin, and I was pretty lousy at following the diet. I hated taking the pills because I knew they would make me feel terrible. I just never felt good.

My company has had a wellness program for about four years. I think we're on our third wellness program now. Back when they started the first program, I decided I'd go to the orientation meeting. The guy speaking reminded me of myself when I was in high school. He was some kind of jock. He said that we would all get some testing, which was basically blood tests, blood pressure, and weight. He also said he wanted us to fill out a health questionnaire.

Several of my fellow employees asked questions but he didn't seem to know much about the medical stuff. Finally someone asked him if this program was mandatory, and he said no. That did it for me. There was no way I wanted my company to know about my health problems. That was my business. In fact, the only people I saw signing up were the young skinny ones.

Then it happened. My CEO called me into his office. He said that my sales numbers had been declining for the last few years and we needed to do something about it. He acknowledged that I had been with the company since it started 25 years ago and that until the last few years, I had been a superstar. He said the company's situation had to change, and I had to change. He gave me a week to come up with a plan and I got the feeling that if he didn't like my plan, he would come up with one of his own.

I was crushed. I went back to my desk and collapsed in my chair. I couldn't catch my breath, and I was sweating a lot. I called my secretary into my office and then felt a pain in my chest. Well, I don't remember much after that until I woke up in the hospital with tubes in my arms and neck, machines beeping, and the doctor and nurse standing next to my bed.

The doctor asked me if I remembered what happened. I said "no." He told me my heart had stopped and they had to restart it. For the first time ever, I was really scared for my life.

According to the doctor, I had an 80% blockage of my coronary arteries and I needed to have heart surgery. When I came out of surgery and woke up, all I could think of was "I'm alive," and seeing the tears in my wife's eyes, I knew she was thinking the same thing.

I went home and felt better than I had for a long time. For one thing, I had some of my old energy back. A week later, during a follow-up appointment, the doctor informed me that my arteries had been slowly closing for many years, which accounted for my fatigue.

He said I would need to continue on all my medications, and he even added some more. I told my doctor how I hated those pills and couldn't imagine living like this until I died. He told me about a local program called 20/20 LifeStyles that had helped many of his patients lose weight and cut down or eliminated their medications. I was ready for anything that would help me feel well again.

I signed up for the 20/20 LifeStyles Program, and my life changed. I may not be 18 years old, but I fit into the same size pants; I'm off all my medications and I have my old energy back. I really feel great. I don't think it's a coincidence that the company's sales were up 11% this year and I got a big bonus. But best of all, I'm the "go to" man again. In fact, I just got finished solving a production problem for our operations VP.

# THE HIDDEN COSTS: PRESENTEEISM, ABSENTEEISM, INDUSTRIAL INJURIES, AND DISABILITY

*Your company's direct healthcare costs are only about 24% of the total cost of employee illness. The following chart displays the total cost of employee health-related expenses[22].*

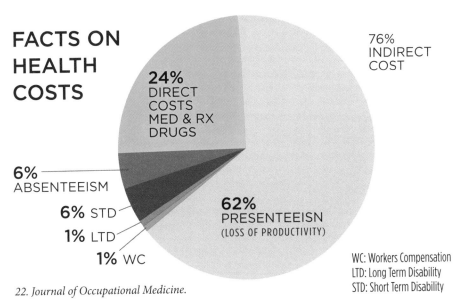

**FACTS ON HEALTH COSTS**

24% DIRECT COSTS MED & RX DRUGS

76% INDIRECT COST

6% ABSENTEEISM

6% STD

1% LTD

1% WC

62% PRESENTEEISN (LOSS OF PRODUCTIVITY)

WC: Workers Compensation
LTD: Long Term Disability
STD: Short Term Disability

22. *Journal of Occupational Medicine.*

As you can see, the indirect costs are actually three times higher than the direct costs of medical treatment and medications. These costs consist of presenteeism, absenteeism, short-term disability, long-term disability, and worker's compensation. All of these "hidden costs" affect your company's bottom line. But the real elephant in the living room is the indirect cost of presenteeism.

Most companies carry a line item in their P & L for medical costs, disability costs, and worker's compensation costs. These numbers are obvious and easy to determine. However, those costs represent only 38% of the total cost.

There are numerous definitions of presenteeism, but they all center on the concept of the employee being at work while impaired by a health issue. The good news is that employees suffering from presenteeism do produce more than those that are completely absent; the bad news is that their productivity suffers substantially. The Harvard Business Review estimates that presenteeism costs companies up to 65% of their TOTAL HEALTHCARE RELATED EXPENSES[23]. These costs are due to reduced productivity, which leads to extra staffing and overtime expenses, loss of sales, poor customer relations, poor employee morale, etc.

But presenteeism isn't easily detected. The employee is still standing or sitting at his/her workstation and usually appears to be functioning. However, that ability to function can be degraded anywhere from 30% to 100%, and there is usually no easy way to detect that.

Many of the medical problems causing presenteeism are very subtle. Some examples are stress, depression, seasonal allergies, migraines, back pain, arthritis, and stomach problems. In these instances the employee usually does not seek medical help and often self-treats the problem or tries to ignore it. But these conditions not only decrease that

23. *Harvard Business Review, "Presenteeism: At Work - But Out of It," October 2004.*

employee's performance, they also affect the performance of all other employees who must interface with the troubled employee.

Sometimes these interface problems are obvious, as when an employee comes to work with a cold or flu and infects other employees. But sometimes it is not obvious, such as when an employee is affected by a high degree of stress or depression or has very low morale.

When individuals are highly stressed, they produce an excess of the hormone cortisol. Cortisol triggers a destructive process that leads to insulin resistance, high cholesterol, weight gain, high blood pressure, type 2 diabetes, and many other disorders. Research has shown that individuals with high stress levels are more contagious than those with a virus. If a highly stressed individual enters an environment (work, home, classroom, etc.), many of those individuals interacting with him begin to show signs of stress and increased cortisol levels within minutes[24].

Absenteeism costs employers an average of $700 per employee per year[25]. That means a company with 500 employees loses $350,000 a year due to absenteeism. That is roughly 1.5% of total payroll. The direct costs for sick pay can be easily determined. However, there are also indirect costs for absenteeism. The indirect costs of overtime, increased head count, and loss of business is NOT part of this $700 per employee per year. Also, since, for a number of reasons managers do not always report employee absenteeism, the total cost of absenteeism is likely higher. Now that I've ruined your day, let's explore what causes absenteeism.

Sixty-six percent (66%) of all absenteeism is due to the illness of the employees or their family. Another 13% is due to "stress,"[26] which makes stress an often overlooked but very costly problem for your company. We will talk about stress a great deal in later chapters.

24. Max Planck Institute for Cognitive and Brain Sciences, 2014.
25. Bureau of Labor Statistics, 2013.
26. American Institute of CPAs, January 17, 2008.

Overweight employees with chronic health conditions, such as diabetes, high cholesterol, and high blood pressure, average between 1.08 and 3.51 sick days per month (over 42 sick days per year), while healthy, normal-weighted employees average .34 days per month (about four days per year)[27]! So this really becomes another added healthcare expense that affects your bottom line.

A study published in the *American Journal of Industrial Medicine*[28] found that individuals with poor aerobic fitness, smokers, individuals with high percent body fat, individuals with high body mass index[29] (BMI), problem drinkers, and individuals with low flexibility were five times more likely to have an industrial injury or an illness than individuals who were physically fit. They further stated that effective industrial injury prevention measures must go beyond job-related risk factors. In order to be effective these measures must address smoking, weight control, and alcohol abuse. In 2010 the cost of industrial injury and illness in the U. S. was $176.9 billion. The average medical cost for an industrial injury was $37,000, and 60 million workdays were lost[30]. Even though the number of industrial injuries is declining, the cost of industrial injuries is increasing. Over the last four years (since the end of the recession) the cost of industrial injuries, for non-construction or manufacturing industries, has risen 26% and is roughly $4,500 per employee per year.

But absenteeism, presenteeism, and industrial injury also have high hidden costs; the costs of extra staffing, short-and long-term disability, hiring and training replacement employees, management and clerical time, and last but not least, workforce morale issues. Issues with absenteeism, presenteeism, and industrial injury cause morale problems

27. *Gallup Well Being, October 17, 2011.*
28. *Personal and non-occupational risk factors and occupational injury/illness, Craig, et. al., American Journal of Industrial Medicine, April 2006.*
29. *Body mass index is a ratio of weight to height. A higher number generally indicates a higher body fat level.*
30. *National Safety Council, Injury Facts, 2012.*

for many reasons. Employees resent having to work harder because their associate isn't working or isn't present. Often times they resent the overtime necessary to cover those who are non-producers. Managers also become over-stressed trying to meet objectives with absent or under-performing subordinates. All of these issues cause morale to worsen; furthermore, worsening morale causes more absenteeism, presenteeism, and industrial injuries. Clearly this is a very damaging vicious cycle.

The math is pretty simple. If you could correct your employee's weight problems and resulting metabolic problems, you could actually reduce your overall payroll costs by 5% to 10%. Clearly the question is how to accomplish that correction.

Many companies have adopted wellness programs in an attempt to reduce or stabilize the direct and indirect healthcare expenses, but the results are less than stellar.

# CHAPTER 3

## WELLNESS BY ATTRACTION

---

## SALES SUPERSTAR

### George - Assistant Sales Manager of a Car Dealership

I was a "car guy." I had been selling cars for over 10 years. I liked what I did and I was good at it. I had been the dealership's top salesman six out of the last eight years. Three years ago I was promoted to an assistant manager position, and since the sales manager was retiring next year, I thought I was the obvious choice.

I work six days a week, usually from noon to closing at 8 p.m. but will stay later if I'm closing a deal. After work, some of the "jocks" would go work out, but I would usually head across the street to the sports bar with some of the other guys for drinks and dinner. About 11 I'd head home, which was only a block-and-a-half away, so I didn't have to drive.

Over the years I had slowly but surely managed to gain about 50 pounds. I didn't like the way I looked, so I had tried a number of diets, but the results were always the same. I would lose five to 10 pounds. But in the next couple of months, I would gain the five or 10 pounds back, and when they came back, they would always bring a few friends.

Our dealership was owned by a man who owned several other dealerships in the area and the owner decided to bring a wellness program into our organization.

The program he chose was called the 20/20 LifeStyles. I was asked to attend a focus group run by one of their staff people but I managed to get out of the group because the timing conflicted with my dinner and drink schedule.

A short time later I attended a mandatory early morning meeting with all the employees at my dealership. The meeting was led by a doctor from the 20/20 LifeStyles Program. I wasn't real happy about this meeting because I wasn't really interested in the wellness program and I really don't do well in the morning.

The doctor talked about the program and told us they would like us all to fill out a health questionnaire, have some testing done.

Our dealership already had a "points" program for providing exceptional customer experience. We could earn points toward gift cards for stores and restaurants. I used all of my gift cards at the sports bar across the street. I really liked the "points" program and was happy and surprised to learn that we could also get points for participating in the wellness program.

I really wanted the points, but I was very uncomfortable with the idea that the company would know all about my health and my weight. I thought being heavy might keep me from getting that sales manager position. I was relieved when the program doctor explained that all health information gathered by the wellness program would be confidential and would not be available to the company. Well, that did it for me, so I signed up.

I completed the questionnaire, had my measurements and blood taken, and caught up on all my vaccinations. Then I met with the doctor to go over my results. The doctor said that my cholesterol levels and blood pressure were too high and that I was 50 pounds overweight. He told me he could refer me to a physician to prescribe medication for my cholesterol and blood pressure issues or he could enroll me in the 20/20

LifeStyles program that was paid by my employer. He explained that he was quite sure that 20/20 LifeStyles would fix my cholesterol and high blood pressure, take off my weight, and give me more energy.

Well, that doctor sure knew what he was talking about. My cholesterol and blood pressure are normal, I lost 56 pounds, and I just ran a 10K race. You guessed it; I've become one of those guys who works out after work instead of hitting the sports bar. Actually, the sports bar group has gotten lots smaller and the workout group larger due to the company's wellness program.

The sales manager met with me a week ago and has started training me to take over his job when he retires. How about that--I work for a great company!

# WHY WELLNESS PROGRAMS DON'T CONTROL HEALTHCARE COSTS

With 88% of employers implementing wellness programs, corporate healthcare costs should be dropping like a rock. But healthcare costs are not dropping--in fact, they're increasing at accelerated rates. There is only one conclusion you can draw from this sad story: MOST CURRENT WELLNESS PROGRAMS DON'T WORK!

A study by the Rand Corporation, sponsored by the U. S. Department of Labor and the U.S. Department of Health and Human services, concluded, "Our statistical analyses suggest that participation in a wellness program over five years is associated with a trend toward lower health care costs and decreasing health care use. We estimate the average annual difference to be $157, but the change is not statistically significant." Looks pretty good until you get to the second sentence; that sentence tells you that the savings are substantially less than the cost of the wellness program, IF SAVINGS REALLY EXIST, and there is no proof that they do exist! They also don't tell us how they "estimated." And guess what, that's the best news out there about wellness programs.

So why don't most wellness programs work? After all, they have the right idea. Sure, it's more cost effective to prevent or cure disease than it is to treat it, but the fault lies in the implementation of the program, which could not be worse. Let's talk about why.

First off, only about half of your employees participate, and does anyone want to guess which half? The healthy half. That's right, these fit people take your incentives because they won't have to do anything to earn it. Most of the employees who know or suspect that they actually have health issues stay away. They don't want to change the unhealthy lifestyles, which have become comfortable for them, and they don't want their peers or managers to know they have health problems. They're afraid that if word got out about their questionable health, the information could affect their jobs or their career path.

On occasion, one of your employees who thinks he is healthy is found to have a chronic illness like diabetes, high blood pressure, or high cholesterol. In that case you've just added another on-going expense to your health care budget. You will be paying for this person's frequent medical appointments, treatments, and medications for the rest of their lives. You'll also pay for the medications for his medication side-effects, etc.

We've all seen drug ads on television. Have you ever noticed the incredibly long list of side-effects and contraindications they read rapidly at the end of the commercial? Did you know that more than 770,000 individuals are hospitalized each year for medical problems arising from medication side effects? There are 4.5 million emergency room, urgent care, and doctor's office visits each year due to medication side effects. Not only that but only 24% of patients on medications take them regularly[31]. Worse, many discontinue taking the medications due to unpleasant side effects and never tell their doctors they have stopped taking them. Many of these patients continue receiving the medications long after they have stopped taking them while you continue to pay for these drugs. Think about it. Do you really want your employees taking more medications?

Also since medications are only treating the symptoms and not changing your employees' or family members' lifestyles, those employees can still go on to have heart attacks, strokes, cancer, etc., and you will have to pay for that as well. Hard to see the savings there.

Second, most wellness programs are coordinated by personal trainers, nutritionists, nurses, or the mysterious "wellness coach." These individuals don't have the background or experience to assess or treat the root causes of illnesses. As we mentioned before, the least expensive medical treatment is the most effective medical treatment. That means it is more cost-effective to send your employee to the best doctor or best hospital, even if the upfront costs are higher. One employee suffering medical complications or needing re-hospitalization will very rapidly eliminate any cost savings you may have obtained by using the cheapest provider for dozens of other employees.

Most wellness programs only provide an online health risk and biometric screening that includes height, weight, blood pressure, blood glucose, and cholesterol levels. When an employee is identified as having a problem, the wellness program provides an "intervention." Some programs will provide a few in-person "counseling" sessions with a "wellness coach" or a few brief telephone contacts with a "health coach[32]," and some may even have luncheon lectures and handouts.

The question remains: is that enough? No. And yet, over *70% of*

31. *US Dept. of Health and Human Services, Agency for Healthcare Research and Quality.*
32. *Most of these "wellness coaches" or "health coaches" are individuals with little or no medical training. Often they are personal trainers with no formal college degree.*

*your healthcare dollars are spent on illnesses that are preventable or curable.* And the shocking truth is that these illnesses are caused by unhealthy lifestyle choices.

So if the brief counseling sessions, phone calls, and online meal trackers worked, your healthcare costs would have gone down 70%. If 70% of these diseases are preventable, why haven't we just prevented them? To fully understand that problem we need to discuss the word "lifestyle."

Your lifestyle is, well, basically everything. It's what time you go to bed at night, what you eat for breakfast, what you do for fun, who your friends are, what beliefs and values you acquired as a child, your religion, the clothes you wear, etc. So it should be no problem to change all that with a phone call or a couple of quick sessions with a "wellness coach," right? WRONG!

If it were easy to change lifestyles, behaviors, and habits, no one would go blind due to type 2 diabetes; no one would have heart attacks at 45 years old due to high cholesterol; no one would have strokes due to high blood pressure related to obesity; no one would smoke; and no one would be an alcoholic or addict. Obviously nobody wants to have these diseases. The difficulty is that since lifestyle is "everything," it's devilishly hard to change. Not only that but lifestyle also has "gravity." What that means is that even if you manage to temporarily change your lifestyle, you will eventually return to your old lifestyle. The reason that happens is because your entire environment hasn't changed. Your spouse still wants to go to that favorite restaurant; your kids want your time, and so does your boss; the doughnut shop is still on your way home from work; your favorite TV show is still on at 11 p.m., etc.

It requires a great deal of effort from a number of very well trained and educated healthcare professionals to change a lifestyle and make it permanent. An employee's current lifestyle needs to be analyzed by a professional who is able to see the truth, even when it is not readily obvious or freely given. Lifestyles, behaviors and habits that have been ingrained over the years need to be changed. The employee's family and/ or support system needs to be addressed. And long-term support needs to be available to counteract the "gravity."

Finally when your employees or their insured family members become ill, have a chronic illness, or get injured on the job, you need a medical expert to supervise their care and make sure they get the very best care.

Let's be honest. Your wellness program simply doesn't offer anything like that.

Still not a believer that the most cost effective medical care is the best medical care? Boeing, Lowe's, and Wal-Mart fly their employees to the Cleveland Clinic for cardiac procedures. Wal-Mart flies them to the Mayo Clinic for transplants. Pepsi flies them to John Hopkins for cardiac procedures and joint replacements. Kroger and CalPERS fly them to the Hoag Orthopedic Institute for orthopedic procedures. These companies even reduce the co-pay if the employee agrees to go to their preferred institution. Does it work? In 2012 Kroger reported that employees who went to their preferred institution cost them 8% less than those who did not. If surgery was involved, the cost was 25.5% less[33]. This was not the result of getting cheaper treatment; it was the result of getting better treatment!

To sum up: you will never begin to control increased healthcare costs by trying to save money on the treatment of medical disorders and diseases. The only way to actually reduce your healthcare costs is by preventing or curing the disease. The good news is that over 70% of those diseases can be prevented or cured.

33. *PwC Health Research Institute, Behind the Numbers 2014*

# CHAPTER 4

## WELLNESS THAT WORKS

---

## MY BODY WAS A TIME BOMB
### *Arthur - Software Engineer at a Large Software Company*

Looking back on it all with what I know now I'm truly amazed that I survived what I put myself through.

There I was, a 26 year-old guy with a good job at a large software company but so completely focused on my work that I didn't understand what the rest of my life was about.

Imagine someone my age who had high blood pressure, extremely high cholesterol, suffered from chronic depression, and weighed 236 pounds. That was me.

To complete that picture, add the fact that I was a heavy smoker. I also consumed literally gallons coffee and diet soda each day, and with all caffeine intake, I was sleeping erratically between two and four hours on weeknights.

I was young and thought I was "bullet proof." That's the way we all lived when I was at college. Bodies were something to be used and abused, and burning the candle at both ends was a way of life.

The stress at work became a huge factor, but more than the stress, it was my lifestyle that had created my sleeplessness.

I considered myself a work-warrior, and I would tough it out while on the job, giving it my all, then I would hit my favorite restaurant on my way home and pig out as a reward for having made it through another long, hard day. No matter how much overtime I worked, I would schedule my departure from the office so that I could get to that restaurant before it closed.

To make things worse, I would never go to sleep until I'd had my fill of video games, which sometimes meant going to bed as early as 10 p.m. and other times as late as 4 a.m. My erratic sleep schedule was constant, but I made it to work on time every morning at 8 a.m.

That was my Monday-through-Friday routine.

On weekends, I was so exhausted that I would spend both days in bed, sleeping 10 or more hours each day to try to make up for the rest of the week. To make things worse, I would frequently buy the largest pizza I could find and have it in bed with me so that I could snack on it whenever I awoke to eat and watch TV.

What truly amazes me about that phase in my life and my deteriorating health is that I didn't consider my lifestyle all that bad. I suppose that was because you never really see how damaging things are until someone who is qualified takes the time to point it out to you.

When I first came to work for my company, I thought I'd check their wellness program out. I went to a talk they gave on nutrition but I was really turned off. They had this really overweight nutritionist, telling us how to eat healthy. Well, I gave up on that idea.

About a year later, my company switched wellness programs, but I had pretty much given up on the idea of a wellness program helping me. Then a couple of guys I worked with went to a talk given by the new 20/20 LifeStyles Wellness Program dietitian and were really impressed, so I attended another talk. I was also impressed by the person giving the talk. He really knew his stuff and could answer any questions that were asked. But more than that it was obvious he "walked the walk" and was really serious about his own health and fitness.

I learned that they could help me change my behavior and my lifestyle. I had tried to change my habits before, but I had always failed. So I signed up for the program.

The doctors at 20/20 LifeStyles, plus my fitness trainer, dietitian, and lifestyle counselors fully understood my problem. They viewed my issues not just as problems with my weight, high cholesterol and high blood pressure, but as lifestyle challenges. They explained that my ongoing depression was related to my lifestyle and life balance. It seemed as if they lived my struggle with me--they were supportive at an emotional level, feeling my pain and celebrating my victories. Their constant care and support had a huge effect, and I began to feel like a different person.

Obviously, the chemical imbalances I created with my addiction to soda, food, and lack of sleep were much to blame for my unhealthy life, and correcting those habits and behaviors certainly meant a lot, but it was the mental change caused by 20/20 LifeStyles that really made the difference.

I began to feel so good about myself that I intuitively didn't want to hurt my body anymore. If you want to call that self-love, I think you can. Initially, I hadn't looked at it that way, but I've since learned that I'm worth it. Keeping the weight off and treating my body with respect is something I continue to do, because it helps me be happy and healthy.

Going forward in my new life, I keep the lessons I learned in the 20/20 LifeStyles program at the top of my mind. I never forget how I was a physical and emotional wreck at 26 years old. And I'll do whatever is necessary to keep my self-respect, self-love, and the respect for my body.

# IF YOU BUILD IT, WILL THEY COME?

No wellness program can work if only half of your employees are involved. As we mentioned before, the employees that do sign up are more likely to be the healthy ones. Remember, *20% of your employees are spending 80% of your healthcare dollars.* What's worse, is that they're costing your company an additional three times as much as you're spending on direct medical care for their presenteeism, absenteeism, worker's compensation, and disability insurance payments[34].

The first step in a plan that really works is getting that 20% who have chronic diseases or risk factors for chronic diseases to participate. Most companies try to do that by offering discounts on health insurance premiums. But clearly that doesn't work.

A good wellness program needs to focus on the "sick" 20%, but it can't stop there. There are other groups that need to be considered. To begin with you must have a program that keeps your healthy employees healthy and prevents them from migrating into the chronic illness group due to unhealthy lifestyles[35].

The program also must help the athletes and weekend warriors in your company. This group can have costly sports injuries due to lack of conditioning, poor form, and poor equipment. And if you insure families, your wellness program needs to be effective for them as well[36].

One last group to consider is employees or family members who are planning to have children. The average cost for a premature birth is $150,000. One day in the neonatal intensive care unit costs $4,500. One out of eight babies is born prematurely, and babies born prematurely continue to have significantly higher medical costs as they grow older.

---

34. *See pie chart page 19.*
35. *Although diabetics make up 9% of your work force, another 20% are following lifestyles that will cause them to become pre-diabetic, which puts them at increased risk for diabetes.*
36. *It is estimated that 40% to 70% of emergency room visits are made by dependents of employees.*

Your wellness company can deliver good prenatal care which can prevent most of these problems and costs.

However, as we mentioned, in order for a wellness program to be successful, your company needs to have a very high rate of participation. The first step in accomplishing this is communicating with your employees in order to find out what they want and don't want in a wellness program. It is especially important that your wellness program contains elements that are attractive to those employees most in need of the program.

Cash is not always king for increasing wellness program participation. There are other techniques, that when executed correctly, have had greater success than reductions in healthcare premium payments and cash incentives. Some non-cash incentives are:

- Name-brand merchandise.
- Gift cards.
- Corporate identified apparel, gym bags, etc.
- Health club memberships.
- Sports equipments such as watches, shoes, heart rate monitors, etc.
- Extra time off.
- Increased contribution to healthcare spending accounts.
- Lower healthcare deductibles or co-pays.

Games are also effective for encouraging participation. Medical information can be difficult and tedious, but games are fun, and everyone likes a competition. Wellness participants can be entered into drawings for prizes based on their entry into the program. You can also have competitions for those employees found to need lifestyle changes to improve their health. And employees can also form teams to compete against each other for rewards and recognition. For games to be effective you must follow some simple guidelines:

- Make the rules simple and consistent.
- Make the game fun and keep it interesting.
- Make it social, so employees can compete or cheer each other on.
- Make game success measurable and update "scores" regularly.

All these techniques have one thing in common: they make wellness program participants an elite group; the participants become special, and everyone likes being special. They also make wellness fun.

Another factor in encouraging employee participation is credibility. Have you ever called your health insurance company to ask about a claim or medication refill? You may have talked to a representative who had little or no knowledge of your condition, had difficulty communicating, and could not even pronounce the name of your condition or medication. Did that leave you with a feeling of confidence? More likely it left you feeling that the phone call was a complete waste of your time and that you would go out of your way to avoid future contact with that insurance company. If your employees' first contact with your wellness program's personnel is similar to that contact with your health insurer, your program has failed even before it got started.

Wellness program personnel MUST be credible. They must fully understand physical illness, emotional illness, nutrition, and exercise, and they must be able to communicate that competence to your employees at their first meeting. This means that instead of having a personal trainer conduct an introductory lecture, you have a physician who is familiar with nutrition and exercise give the employees their orientation. And every single provider in the wellness program chain must also be competent; this includes the person answering the phone or the person drawing blood for labs. When your employee asks a question, the answer should never be "I don't know" or worse yet a made-up answer to conceal a lack of knowledge. Your employees may not be medical doctors or Ph.D.'s, but they can tell a provider who knows what he or she is talking about from one who is "winging it."

Some other reasons why employees do not participate in wellness programs are:

- They do not want their employer to know about their medical or emotional condition. They feel it might make it more difficult for them to progress in the company.

- They are in denial of the true nature of their health. Denial is a comfortable place. It prevents the stress and anxiety that might occur if an individual were to confront the fact that they are NOT healthy.

- Employees may want to hide their physical condition from their spouse. There are numerous reasons for this, such as not wanting them to be worried, not wanting to be "nagged" about it, or not wanting their spouse to think less of them.

- They may also not want their co-workers to know that they have health issues. Medical issues can be embarrassing, and the opinion of one's peers is important. Sexual disorders, alcohol or drug use disorders, emotional disorders, and even disorders such as obesity or diabetes can be embarrassing.

To sum it up, before your wellness program can be effective, you need a very high rate of employee and employee's family participation. You must communicate with your employees to develop a wellness program that has advantages for a wide range of your employees and their families--everyone from the athlete to the chronically ill. Furthermore, you must do it in a way that makes the employee want to be part of the program and makes it fun. Your wellness providers need to be competent, professional, personable, and they must be able to deal with the many reasons employees reject wellness programs

# CHAPTER 5

## THE BUILDING BLOCKS

---

## SLOWING DOWN A BIT
### *Phyllis - Executive Assistant for a Manufacturing Company*

I had worked for the company for 24 years. I started out in the mailroom, and for the last 10 years, I had been the executive assistant to the vice president of operations. My two children were grown; I had great kids, and I was as proud as any mom could be.

But then, as I got a bit older, and with the kids gone, I had lost a sense of who I was. All my life I had been the caregiver; I took care of everything for my boss, my husband, and my kids. But with only my husband, Al, to care for at home, I felt lost.

Don't get me wrong, my husband is a great guy, but he has his career, his friends, and his Monday night football. But, other than work, I didn't seem to have much.

I had noticed that I seemed tired all the time, that my skin was really dry and that I was cold all the time. I just thought this was part of getting older.

My company announced they would be starting a wellness program and had contracted with the 20/20 LifeStyles Wellness Program to provide services. I knew that my company was struggling to control healthcare costs and thought this was an approach worth trying. Also, my own cost-sharing expenses for the company-sponsored health insurance plan were rising every year, and I hoped the wellness approach could help with that too.

The first thing the wellness program provider wanted to do was hold several focus groups with our employees to find out our needs. I was asked by my boss to set up these groups. I followed up with several of our employees who had attended the groups, and I was impressed with their positive opinions about the experience. I thought, "Maybe these guys know what they're doing."

The next step in the process was several "brown bag" lunch introductory lectures. I had to arrange those as well and took the opportunity to attend a couple. At the same time 20/20 LifeStyles had us fill out a questionnaire that included a "lifestyle history" and had a person on site measuring biometrics and drawing blood. On the questionnaire I answered yes to being cold a lot, to having dry skin and to feeling tired a lot.

The program also had someone come to our office and discuss the testing results with each of us. When I went to talk to this person about my results, I was really surprised to discover that he was a doctor and had already studied my report. I told him I had always maintained my normal body weight, but that I would occasionally gain 10-15 pounds but then would diet and get back to normal. He told me all of my blood tests were normal except for my thyroid test. He said normally they don't test thyroid function but since I reported fatigue, dry skin and feeling cold all the time on the questionnaire, they included that test. He said that the thyroid problem was easily corrected with medication and in a few weeks those symptoms would go away.

The doctor seemed like someone I could trust, so when he asked me to come into the 20/20 LifeStyles performance lab, I agreed.

When I went they measured my body fat using dual x-ray absorptiometry, or DEXA. The 20/20 LifeStyles doctor explained that the very low-powered x-ray machine was the only way to accurately measure percent of total body fat. The doctor then informed me that my body fat was 44% and normal for me would be 27% to 31%, which placed me in the obese category even though my body weight and BMI were normal. He explained how gaining weight and then losing it with fad diets often stripped a body of muscle and replaced it with fat.

I was a believer! I would do anything he told me to do, and I did. The company paid for me to have an exercise physiologist set me up on a fitness program. It wasn't easy. I got up an hour early five days a week and worked out at their gym. The company also paid for me to meet with a dietitian every other week.

With the thyroid medicine, the exercise and learning how to eat healthy, I lost 20 pounds of fat and replaced it with 6 pounds of muscle. My body fat is now 25%, I am a size-six dress, and I can go all day without getting tired. As added bonuses my skin is great, I'm not cold all the time, and I am sleeping better than I have since I was 12.

My husband is thrilled and we've started bicycling together on the weekends. I am taking on new responsibilities at work, and the other day my boss asked me what had happened to me. I answered, "Wellness!"

## WELLNESS THAT WORKS

Phyllis' story is a result of a wellness program that works.

Phyllis has her energy back, looks great, and feels great. Her employer retained a valuable employee, and she has become even more valuable. Good wellness programs are a win-win for everyone. Unfortunately, most wellness programs don't deliver. Why? Because it takes a lot of expertise to create a GOOD wellness program. It doesn't take much to administer a health risk questionnaire and collect biometrics. Just about any provider can do that. But that just isn't nearly enough!

Here are the four P's of a good wellness program:

- Participation
- Probing analysis of the data
- Prevention
- Programs to successfully deal with health issues

In Chapter Four, we discussed the need for a high rate of participation. Without this, no wellness program can be successful in reducing corporate health insurance costs. But participation alone does not guarantee a successful program.

Health risk questionnaires and biometrics provide useful information, but without an intelligent, probing analysis of this data, too many of your employees will slip through the cracks. Phyllis is a good example. Most wellness programs would have looked at her health risk questionnaire and biometrics and conclude that she was at normal weight and had no health risks. She might have been advised to exercise and modify her diet slightly. This would have been done by a phone call or letter from a person she had never met. The person initiating the call or letter would have been a personal trainer or technician. As a result, Phyllis' fatigue, skin problems and coldness would have continued and due to her high percent of body fat she might have developed metabolic disorders like diabetes, stroke or heart attack.

In addition to a health risk questionnaire, it is important to administer a lifestyle questionnaire. Trying to interpret biometrics without awareness of an individual's lifestyle is like finding an address without a map. You know the numbers, but you don't have the context to fully interpret them. It is important to have all the information and have a provider who can interpret that information correctly. Furthermore, that information should be provided to the employee by knowledgeable medical provider. Without the provider's personal touch and credibility, it is likely the employee will ignore the advice.

Next we need to consider how a wellness program can stop health problems before they start. Prevention is a critical component of a wellness program. In fact, preventions is the key to long-term healthcare cost containment. Prevention efforts are geared in two directions. The first is preventing your healthy employees from becoming sick employees. The second is preventing your employees with risk factors from developing chronic illnesses.

Healthy employees need to understand nutrition, exercise, and stress-coping techniques. These are vital for health maintenance. Employees also must learn healthy eating. Furthermore they must also learn to cope with stress to avoid producing stress hormones that lead to metabolic disorders. Finally, they need to learn when to see a doctor and when they don't need to see a doctor.

The problem is that your healthy employees are, well, healthy. They just don't think they need health guidance. It's important that your wellness provider has staff that can connect with this segment. This takes individuals with credibility who are knowledgeable about the activities that your healthy employees enjoy.

The second segment in this "healthy" group are "the ticking time bombs." These employees already have risk factors, which, if left untreated, will lead to catastrophic diseases. What's more, their productivity may already be declining, due to frequent illnesses and a high degree of presenteeism and absenteeism. Left untreated, this group has a very high probability of developing chronic diseases like diabetes, hypertension, heart disease, and other metabolic disorders. Your wellness program must identify these employees and treat them, and it is essential that their treatment be effective.

The last group we have to consider are those individuals who already have chronic diseases. Clearly these individuals are the 20% who are spending 80% of your healthcare dollars. They are the group that is costing you the most in lost productivity due to presenteeism and absenteeism. They are the group that is running up your disability costs. Clearly any improvement made in the health of these individuals will make a big impact on your bottom line. To deal effectively with this group, your wellness provider must be able to reverse these diseases and disorders where possible and where not possible, to manage them using the most effective medical providers and therapies. Obviously, successfully managing this group takes a high level of skill and medical sophistication.

In 2006 overweight and obesity-related illnesses cost corporations 12.9% of all their healthcare dollars, and without doubt that figure is significantly higher now due to the ever- increasing rates of overweight and obesity. The mandatory preventive care portion of the ACA requires that all these individuals receive screening and counseling for this condition[37]. The problem is that fewer than 2% of those who lose weight are able to maintain that weight loss. This figure includes all national weight loss programs, medical programs, and drug therapies. Your wellness program needs to do much better than this dismal statistic.

There are two other topics that can have a major impact on your healthcare spending and your bottom line. These topics are pregnancy/childbirth and vaccination.

You may remember that a number of years ago there was an Academy Award winning movie called *Million Dollar Baby*. Million dollar babies do occur, and they will not win any awards for your company. Recently, we talked to one company that had a problem-pregnancy and birth. The mother was hospitalized for six weeks prior to delivery. She had several medical procedures during that time to avoid

37. See Appendix A.

a severely premature birth. She delivered the baby after only 26 weeks of gestation. The baby was treated in the neonatal intensive care unit for 16 weeks and needed several medical procedures. The result was an 878,000-dollar baby. Not quite a million, but guess what, the mother (spouse of the employee) is pregnant again. Much of this expense can be prevented with an adequate pregnancy program that starts before the mother gets pregnant and ends after the baby is delivered and the mother is restored to her optimal fitness.

Less than half of your employees and their families are adequately vaccinated. Myths and outright lies have caused people to be anxious about vaccination. Having a high percentage of your employees and their families adequately vaccinated is a very inexpensive method of preventing serious illness and saving healthcare dollars. Your wellness program not only needs to provide vaccinations but must provide education and incentives to employees to overcome the fear caused by misinformation and ignorance. Once again, this requires credibility on the part of your wellness provider's staff. See appendix C for recommended vaccination schedules.

It's time to ask yourself: how well does your wellness program perform on these difficult and complex issues?

# CHAPTER 6

## THE 20/20 LIFESTYLES WELLNESS PROGRAM

---

## FIXING THE SYMPTOMS
### *Kyle - Partner in a Large Tech Company*

I had become the great rationalizer. Things that I wouldn't accept ten years ago seemed perfectly normal to me. My two best friends were rationalization and denial. I was 51 years old and at the peak of my career. I worked for a well-known tech company and had just been promoted to "partner," a very high level in the company. I was in charge of a team of 225 software professionals and was considered a rising star in my company. Unfortunately my star wasn't the only thing that was rising. My belt size and weight were rising right along with it. But I rationalized that I was okay, because I worked very hard, and in my time off I tried to be a good father to my two teenage sons and a good husband to my wife. It's kind of amazing to me now that my rationalization and denial allowed me to ignore the fact that at 310 pounds, I was a health disaster waiting to happen.

I wasn't blind, I knew I wasn't an example of fitness or health by any means, but I had accepted who I was physically. I was a guy who exercised a little once in a while, like playing golf. I thought of myself as someone who enjoyed his free time, which meant eating and drinking everything I wanted, when I wanted.

My company had started a wellness program a few years back, but I avoided it like the plague. My excuse was that I didn't have time for it, but the reality was that I really didn't want to hear the bad news. The problem was, now that I was a "partner" it was mandatory that I have an "executive physical," and guess who did the executive physicals: the 20/20 LifeStyles Wellness Program. The physical itself went very well. The staff was very efficient, I didn't have to sit in a waiting room for more than a couple of minutes, and they did a very thorough assessment of my health.

That was the good news. Two days after my physical, one of their doctors sat down with me, and that's when the bad news began. The doctor said I had type 2 diabetes, stroke- level high blood pressure, high triglycerides, and very high cholesterol. He said I was very lucky that I had come in for the physical and told me that if I didn't deal with these health issues, the probability of my reaching 60 was pretty small.

He told me he could refer me to a doctor to place me on medications for diabetes, hypertension, and high cholesterol, or I could enter into the 20/20 LifeStyles Program, which was covered by my company's wellness plan. He said he felt there was an excellent chance the program could normalize my health issues without medications.

The doctor explained the program to me and told me it was my choice. He was very professional and seemed quite caring, but I still wasn't ready to make a decision. All of my rationalization and denial had collapsed, and I was in shock. I didn't know what to think.

I had read about some of those medications: statins like Lipitor, blood pressure meds like Lasix, and of course, the eventuality of insulin injections and all the related health issues brought on by diabetes including Alzheimer's disease. What became obvious was that my life was about to become one large prescription of daily medications, compounded by all their side effects like muscle aches, nausea, and dizziness. Recently there's even been evidence that Lipitor, used long term, can cause breast cancer and diabetes--a disease I wanted to cure.

The worst part was the medications didn't cure the disease, they just fixed the symptoms.

That night all I could think about was my father and his health problems. It seemed like my dad had doctor appointments every week. He went blind and wound up in a wheelchair when he was 56 and died when he was 59.

That really scared me and I didn't sleep very well that night. The next day at work I had difficulty concentrating and wasn't really all there. I was suprised when I got a call from the wellness program doctor that afternoon. He seemed to know how distressed I was and asked if I had made a decision. That did it for me. I didn't want to start taking all those medications, and I didn't want to die young. I told him to sign me up.

I went to the introductory seminar given by Dr. Dedomenico and discovered a new hope. 20/20 LifeStyles was so much more than just a diet. It was a complete lifestyle program that was run by highly skilled doctors, psychologists, dietitians, and exercise physiologists. My shock and depression turned into excitement and hope. I was totally ready. I never missed a meeting, an appointment, or a workout for the entire length of the program.

That decision saved my life! Not only did it save my life but it also gave me back the high quality life that I used to enjoy.

I've always been a results-oriented guy, so I'll cut to the outcome. I lost 120 pounds, I CURED my diabetes, I have the blood pressure of a 20 year-old, and my triglycerides and cholesterol levels are super low.

But that's not the half of it. My exercise physiologist was a marathoner, and he actually ran a 5K and 10K race with me. I found with all my new energy and endurance that I truly loved running. So I entered a couple of half-marathons and then ran some full marathons. Much to my surprise, I found I was a really good runner and actually had some times under three-and-a-half hours.

My work group was so amazed when I told them that I had qualified for the Boston Marathon, they took up a collection to fly some of my work associates to Boston to cheer for me. I've started a running group at work, and last week we had almost 50 people show up for our lunchtime run.

All this from an ex-310-pound heart attack waiting to happen. My company and the 20/20 LifeStyles Wellness Program have turned me into a walking (running?) miracle.

## WELLNESS PROGRAM ROI?

Every successful business is deadly serious about ROI. They examine overall return in addition to division and department returns. If a business unit is not producing a return, it must be corrected or eliminated. These are business facts of life.

But for some reason, these facts do not apply to wellness programs. It is accepted that wellness programs are necessary and there is some vague belief that they will help moderate the increase in healthcare costs. And yet, no one calculates the ROI. We suspect the reason for this is that no one really believes there is a return on the cost of the investment made in wellness programs.

But let's take a look at Kyle. Clearly Kyle was a valued and important asset to his company. That was indicated when he was promoted to "partner." But Kyle was going to cost the company a great deal of money due to his metabolic disorders. The average cost (direct and indirect) of treating employees who have high cholesterol is $5,400 per year[38], hypertension $4,100 per year, and type 2 diabetes a whopping $13,700 per year. That adds up to $23,200 per year, every year, for

---

38. *American Diabetes Association.*

the rest of Kyle's life. If Kyle sees the same physician to treat all of his metabolic disorders, the yearly cost might be reduced by a few thousand dollars. However, Kyle's metabolic disorders make him a prime candidate for stroke, heart attack, kidney failure, blindness, or one of the many complications of these conditions. At that point, Kyle's employer is not only looking at the loss of Kyle's productivity, the employer will also have to foot the bill for hundreds of thousands of dollars of tests, procedures, hospitalizations, surgeries, and rehabilitation.

20/20 LifeStyles placed Kyle in a 44-week program because his BMI was calculated to be 41. The cost of Kyle's 20/20 LifeStyles program was $12,680. Kyle's program had a ROI of seven months. That means Kyle's program paid for itself in seven months, plus the company will continue to save between $20,000 and $23,000 every year. If you like the idea of assessing your wellness program using ROI as a criterion, read on.

Many companies feel wellness programs are a benefit when it comes to hiring high quality employees. These programs also boost employee morale and company loyalty. We agree that those benefits are important, but we feel that the main benefit of wellness programs must be the reduction of direct and indirect healthcare costs. Kyle's story is a very good example of that. Not only did the 20/20 LifeStyles Wellness Program produce an impressive ROI, it also greatly increased Kyle's loyalty and gratitude to the company. Furthermore it improved the morale of his work group and running group. In fact, we would propose that any wellness program would have to do all this to really be effective.

# COMPETENCE & PROFESSIONALISM ARE THE KEYS

Kyle was in strong denial about his health. We mentioned earlier that 20% of your employees spend 80% of your healthcare dollars and those 20% are usually in denial. What shocked Kyle out of his denial was the competence of the doctor whom Kyle met at the 20/20 LifeStyles Wellness Program. But had that doctor not called him at work the next day, Kyle still may have slipped back into his denial and suffered the serious health consequences of that denial. It was the competence and the professionalism of the 20/20 LifeStyles physician that made the difference to Kyle and to his company.

The key is competence! The professionals presenting the brown bag lunches, the staff gathering the biometrics, and the physicians presenting the biometric results to your employees must all create an environment that strongly encourages and validates program participation. When it comes to healthcare, we all want our providers to be the very best.

When Kyle participated in the 20/20 LifeStyles Program he found competence in depth. Not only were those professionals who worked with his company competent but, also all of the program people he had contact with were highly skilled. Let's look at what that means.

When Kyle called to schedule an intake appointment with the 20/20 LifeStyles program, he first spoke to a receptionist. He was not placed on hold and did not have to go through a telephone tree to talk to her. The receptionist took his information in an intelligent, professional manner and transferred that information to the intake coordinator. The intake coordinator had the staff availability at her fingertips and in a matter of minutes was able to schedule all of Kyle's appointments at times that were convenient for him.

Kyle then came in for his first appointment and quickly realized that every member the staff who would be working with him "walked the walk." They were all professionals who were not only skilled in their areas of expertise, they were excited about their own health and fitness. They became Kyle's role models.

Kyle totally trusted his doctor, exercise physiologist, dietitian, and lifestyle counselor because of their competence and their personal love of health and fitness. For those reasons, he wanted to be like them, and that led him to succeed.

Competence and professionalism are the keys to attracting employees to the program and making them successful in the program. These qualities need to be seamless throughout your employees' experience with your wellness program.

Be sure your current wellness program provides these most important qualities.

# CHAPTER 7

## ELEMENTS OF THE
## 20/20 LIFESTYLES PROGRAM

### MY POOR WIFE
*Darren - IT Manager for a CPA Firm*

I was 44 year-old IT Manager for a moderately sized CPA firm. I loved my job, and my company was a great place to work. I really didn't want to leave the company, but my situation at home was making it look like that's exactly what I'd have to do. You see, my wife Laura, who is only 37, had severe fibromyalgia. Her fibromyalgia pain was so bad that most nights she had problems sleeping. Of course that meant I didn't get much sleep either. I love my wife very much, and her agony broke my heart.

We had tried everything to control her pain and had gone to many doctors, naturopaths, chiropractors, and anyone else who said they could help her. She was taking a number of medications and had severe side effects from some of them. Just last year, one of the medications that actually seemed to help a bit caused her to develop a bleeding ulcer. Of course, she had to stop taking it.

On the days when Laura was so completely disabled, I had to stay home, get the kids to school, and take care of Laura. The problem was that those days were getting more frequent, and it began to look like I would soon have to get a job where I could work from home.

About a year and a half ago, my company started using the 20/20 LifeStyles Wellness Program. 20/20 LifeStyles really stressed that managers needed to set a good example by participating in the program. As I said, I liked my company and always tried to be a team player, so I signed up for the program.

I attended a couple of talks and during one of them, the 20/20 LifeStyles doctor, who was giving the presentation, mentioned that fibromyalgia was a metabolic disorder and that the program treated metabolic disorders. After the talk, I asked the doctor if he could talk to me for a few minutes. He was happy to do so, and so I asked him about my wife. I was very impressed with his knowledge about her condition.

When I mentioned Laura having tried a drug that had helped, but caused her problems, he said, "There have been quite a number of side effects with that medication. By the way, did she develop an ulcer or any other stomach problems?"

Well, I was pretty amazed. He suggested that Laura come visit him at his office and bring her history of procedures, tests, and medications along.

At the conclusion of Laura's appointment, the program doctor told Laura that he thought he could help her. 20/20 LifeStyles had a version of the metabolic disorder module that they used to treat fibromyalgia. The good news was they didn't use drugs or medical procedures in their treatment.

When I came home that night and Laura told me what the doctor had said, I felt a bit of hope. Neither of us was terribly excited because we had tried so many things before with no relief. But we both had a really good feeling about that doctor and the 20/20 program in general.

Well, Laura was in the program for almost six months, and there were days at the beginning that were pretty difficult. The exercise took a lot of effort, and she was sometimes pretty uncomfortable, but the 20/20 LifeStyle staff had answers that always helped her to feel better and get past the rough spots. After a difficult day, they would always call her at home that evening to see how she was doing.

That was about a year-and-a-half ago. Today, my wife, our kids, and I enjoy bicycle riding in the summer and skiing in the winter. Laura has her full mobility back, and as long as she keeps to her exercise schedule and nutrition plan, she is completely pain-free. Not only that but she is off all medications.

When somebody saves someone you love, there is almost no way special enough to express your gratitude. So when they asked me to tell our story, I said "absolutely."

# A COMPREHENSIVE PROGRAM

The point we are trying to make with Darren's story is that your wellness program must be expert at treating a wide variety of conditions and people--and they must be able to show results. Laura's disabling fibromyalgia at 37 years of age is not a common condition, but 20/20 LifeStyles has treated it many times before and has perfected a treatment module that works exceedingly well. A wellness program that really works must be able to successfully treat:

- Overweight and obesity
- High cholesterol levels
- High blood pressure
- Diabetes type 2
- Heart disease
- Kidney disease
- Osteoarthritis
- Fibromyalgia
- Chronic fatigue syndrome
- Stress

- Depression
- Sleep disorders
- Acute back problems
- Alcohol and drug addiction
- Vaccinations for seasonal, lifetime, and overseas travel
- Pregnancy and healthy baby programs
- Financial problems
- Ergonomic issues
- Allergies
- Headaches
- Gastrointestinal problems

Plus this program must be able to manage chronic disease, surgeries, and medical procedures to ensure that your employee gets the best treatment (which is also the most cost-effective treatment). And they must do all of these things well.

If you think that's a tall order, perhaps that's why your current or past wellness programs have not led to a reduction in your medical costs.

## ONE SIZE DOESN'T FIT ALL

Most wellness companies offer you a choice of some pre-designed programs. These programs were NOT designed specifically for your company. Since all companies are different, a properly developed wellness program needs to be designed within the framework of your company's management goals and employee composition. It must also be able to address the needs of insured family members.

So the first step in setting up a wellness program should always be a meeting with your company's management to mutually develop goals that will lead to successfully controlling your healthcare costs, while simultaneously improving productivity, loyalty, and employee morale.

Once that step is complete, the wellness company needs to get to know your employees. In the 20/20 LifeStyles Wellness Program, we do this by conducting several focus groups with a range of employees and their spouses. Once we have that data, we again meet with management to discuss a program specifically designed for their company.

Based on our knowledge of that company, we begin a program that will eventually enroll up to 80% or more of the company's employees. We specifically target those who have chronic diseases or risk factors for chronic diseases. Remember, one of the main reasons most wellness programs don't work is poor employee participation rates.

To achieve this level of participation, we heavily promote the program. We present lectures on topics such as Coping with Stress, Why Vaccinate, Healthy Mom-Healthy Baby, High Blood Pressure and High Cholesterol, Curing Type 2 Diabetes, Sleeping Better, Problems with Alcohol and Drugs, and many more.

In the 20/20 LifeStyles Wellness Program we ensure that all staff interfacing with a company's employees will be well-educated, well-spoken professionals who are themselves examples of living a healthy lifestyle.

Like other wellness programs, we bulk email employees and provide pamphlets for companies to distribute. But we understand this is not enough to get the level of employee participation necessary for a successful wellness program. Having met with your employees we are able to build a strategic recruitment plan based on your company and your employees. We also feel it is vital for all management personnel to participate in the program. We have found that without management participation, the program will have only limited success.

The next step for our program is to have each employee fill out our on-line health and lifestyles survey. Then, a trained 20/20 LifeStyles staff person takes weights, measurements, and draws blood. Blood tests may vary from employee to employee based on survey data and measurements. For example, if an employee has an elevated BMI and had mentioned fatigue in the survey, thyroid tests would also be run on the blood sample. The 20/20 LifeStyles Wellness Program is always designed specifically for each individual employee.

After these initial steps, our medical doctor then presents each employee's results in a face-to-face meeting. At that time the employee is given treatment recommendations and options. Employees with no health issues or risks can use this time to ask health, fitness, and lifestyle questions.

Those employees with risk factors or disorders are offered a program designed to correct the problem. These programs are individually designed to meet the employee's needs.

Let's use Darren as an example. Darren participated in the program because he was a group manager, and we stressed the need for management to set an example by their participation. When he sat down with our doctor, he learned that 20/20 LifeStyles was very familiar with fibromyalgia and had excellent success in treating it. The program did not rely on multiple medications and their unpleasant and dangerous side effects. Darren and Laura were given an option that could avoid the medications, tests, procedures, and surgeries. Laura's talks with our doctor made her decision easy.

Well, you know the rest of Darren's story, and it certainly has a very happy ending for both Darren and Laura. Laura got to be pain free and enjoy her life and her family; Darren got to keep the job that he loved. The company got to stop paying for tests, procedures, medications, and the eventual surgeries that Laura would have had. Everybody won.

# CHAPTER 8

## 20/20 LIFESTYLES
## PREVENTION MODULES

Since 80% of your healthcare dollars are spent on 20% of the individuals in your insurance plan, it's important that your wellness program be able to identify those who are healthy, those with risk factors for serious illness, and those with chronic illnesses. An employer is not allowed to have access to this information. However, employees may still be very guarded about their health information because they fear that this information will affect their employment or advancement with the company. Your wellness company must work very hard to win the trust of your company's employees.

Our prevention modules work in two ways. First they help employees live healthier lifestyles, thus avoiding costly illnesses and injuries. Second they allow an interface between the 20/20 LifeStyles Wellness Program and the employees which then develops into a trusting relationship.

## EMPLOYEE RECRUITING

As we have stated several times, no wellness program can work if the percentage of participating employees is too small. The 20/20 LifeStyles Wellness Program developed an "Incentive Point" system for encouraging participation. We have found that when this is done correctly, you can expect up to 80% of your employees to participate in the program. This is how the Incentive Point system works:

70

The system gives employees Incentive Points for complying with each specific task in the 20/20 LifeStyles program. Points are assigned a nominal cash value that can be used to calculate rewards. For example if you assign a nominal cash value of $0.10 per point, a $50 gift card would require the employee to redeem 500 Incentive Points. This system is basically the same system that was initiated by United Airlines (and copied by all other airlines). The system was hugely successful for United and has been adopted by hotel chains, car rental agencies, and credit card companies. It is a proven motivational system.

These incentive points are given to employees for each step in participating in the wellness program, and the number of points for each step is weighted depending on the importance of that step for the success of the program. For example, you might give all employees 1000 points for completing the online health and lifestyle questionnaire and getting their biometrics measured. But you might give them 1500 incentive points for successfully completing a smoking cessation module and another 1500 incentive points for remaining nicotine free for an additional year.

The point value of each step is something that you can change depending on the goals and needs of the company. However the rewards you establish that are redeemed for points need to be items that appeal to a wide cross section of your employees and their families.

We have found that the following steps need to be rewarded for the program to be most successful.

- Completing the online health and lifestyle survey.
- Completing biometric measurement and testing.
- Having all required vaccinations.
- Watching educational videos online.
- Attending and/or online viewing wellness talks.
- Successfully completing necessary treatment modules.

- Using health insurance benefits only for preventive care for one year.
- Having perfect attendance.

There are many others that can be added to the list depending on your company's goals and needs.

# BIOMETRIC SCREENING

Almost every wellness program provides biometric screening. However, 20/20 LifeStyles performs what we call "intelligent biometric screening" that is modified to meet the needs of the individual employee. Based on the employee's responses to the online health and lifestyle questionnaire and their other biometric data, additional tests may be performed. Furthermore, the employee does not get a letter informing them of their results; instead, the employee actually sits down with a physician to discuss their results and his or her options. Naturally all individually identifiable questionnaire and biometric data are held confidential by the 20/20 LifeStyles Program. Below are the specifics of the biometric program:

1. Weight/Height to determine BMI (body mass index).
2. Waist circumference if indicated by BMI.
3. Blood Pressure.
4. Blood draw for:
   a. Cholesterol screening (LDL, HDL, Ratio, Triglycerides).
   b. Serum glucose.
5. Blood draw for HbA1C (for diagnosis of blood sugar problems) if:
   a. Health questionnaire indicates.
   b. Serum glucose is over 100.
   c. Patient is pre-diabetic or diabetic.

6. Blood draw for TSH (for diagnosis of thyroid problems) if:
    a. Health questionnaire indicates.
    b. Patient is obese.
    c. Patient is known to be hypothyroid.
    d. Patient relates hypothyroid symptoms to biometric testing staff.
7. Blood sample for vitamin D if:
    a. Health and lifestyle questionnaire indicates.
    b. Individual is over 40 years of age.
8. Additional blood samples if:
    a. Individual has known liver disease.
    b. Individual has known kidney disease.
    c. Individual is taking prescription drugs known to cause vitamin deficiencies, e.g.: Prilosec causes vitamin D deficiency.
9. Confidential in-person consultation with physician on:
    a. Results of health and lifestyles survey.
    b. Results of biometric data and blood tests.
    c. Recommended vaccinations.
10. A follow-up letter from 20/20 physician to employee or family member after in-person consultation.
    a. Outlining any disorders diagnosed.
    b. Outlining corporate support available.
    c. Providing employee with name/number of 20/20 contact.
11. Transmittal of the employee's or family member's evaluation to their primary care physician.
    a. Summary of tests.
    b. Copy of the follow-up letter.

# EMPLOYEE EDUCATION

This section presents a wide-range of modules designed to keep your employees and their families healthy. It is very important that your wellness company informs your employees and insured families as to what they can do to stay healthy and live quality lives. We use brown bag talks to educate employees on how to avoid developing diseases and disorders and lead healthy lives. These talks can be delivered as a combination of brown bag lunch talks and short talks during department meetings. This information needs to be presented to your employees by knowledgeable, personable, and credible professionals. Talks usually last from 20 to 30 minutes and include time for questions and answers. These talks can include:

- Why it's important to fill out the health and lifestyle questionnaire and have biometrics performed.
- The phony vaccine scare-why vaccinate.
- Managing family finances.
- Personal ergonomics at work and at home.
- Assertiveness and boundary setting.
- Nutritional supplements, what do I need.
- Quick and easy healthy cooking.
- Work/life balance.
- How to control stress.
- Managing depression.
- Parenting for the working family.
- Principles of healthy relationships.
- Self-talk and self-love: stop blaming and start accepting.
- Introduction to fitness.
- Diet and wellness.
- Dealing with foot, leg, and back pain.
- How to save money using generic versus brand name medications.

- Preventing breast cancer.
- The food/mood connection.
- Staying sharp and exercising your brain.
- Managing emotions in the workplace.
- Holiday eating and drinking.
- How to sleep better.
- So you want to have a baby.
- Managing your weight.
- When you need the emergency room or urgent care and when you don't.

We understand you will be limited in how many of these talks you can schedule each year. If you can provide your employees with five to ten talks per year, that would be very helpful. We have been successful at scheduling these talks during the last 20 minutes of department meetings or at lunchtime as a brown bag lunch series. We strongly recommend the use of incentive points to encourage attendance at these talks. We also have these talks available as online videos for viewing by family members.

Once again, the quality of the individual providing the talks is all-important. Knowledgeable, professional, and charismatic presenters will go a long way toward encouraging your employees and insured family members to begin focusing on their health and the health of their families. This attitude change will result in healthier employees, healthier family members, and medical cost savings for the company.

For employees and families who desire more information on a topic or prefer to view an online video presentation about a topic, we offer over 45 videos for viewing. These videos are about 20 minutes in length and are continuously updated with new research and state-of-the-art information. This is our current list of videos, but new and updated videos are added on a regular basis:

- 20/20 LifeStyles Intro Seminar 1
  - Weight gain is not your fault. Meet Dr. Mark Dedomenico and learn the key contributors to weight gain.
- 20/20 LifeStyles Intro Seminar 2
  - Learn more about the reasons for weight gain, including the hormone ghrelin, which sends you searching for food.
- 20/20 LifeStyles Intro Seminar 3
  - Find out about the hormone leptin, a long-term regulator of food intake, and how being insulin resistant can lead to weight gain.
- 20/20 LifeStyles Intro Seminar 4
  - Discover how insulin resistance affects the body, what your set point is, and how Non-Exercise Activity Thermogenesis (NEAT) is an important part of weight loss.
- 20/20 LifeStyles Intro Seminar 5
  - Did you know sugar causes the release of a chemical to your brain's reward center? Learn about Reward Center eating and how to create a healthier lifestyle.
- 20/20 LifeStyles Intro Seminar 6
  - Get started with the 20/20 LifeStyles program and our uniquely successful approach to permanent weight loss.
- Exercising and Having Fun
  - Do you dread the word exercise? You'll learn how to create an exercise plan that is fun and understand the health benefits of being active.
- Coping with Celebration
  - Do you find yourself falling off plan during holidays and celebrations? Learn useful tips and tricks to help you maintain your new healthy lifestyle.

- Grocery Shopping 1
  - Rediscover the produce section and receive a variety of smart shopping tips.
- Grocery Shopping 2
  - Find out why healthy protein sources are an indispensable part of your weight-loss plan.
- Grocery Shopping 3
  - Get the scoop on which healthy fats and grains to pick up at the grocery store.
- Grocery Shopping 4
  - Learn how to decipher food labels. Find out what's hiding in the health food section.
- Creating Healthy Family Lifestyles Habits
  - Discover the key factors in developing and maintaining a healthy lifestyle for you and your family. Learn what causes children to be overweight.
- Metabolism and NEAT
  - Get the details on Non-Exercise Activity Thermogenesis (NEAT). Find out how NEAT can improve your chances of losing weight.
- Misconceptions About Dieting
  - Get the truth about common dieting and exercise myths.
- Planning Around Temptation
  - Do you struggle to make healthy choices at fast-food restaurants, parties, and snack time? Learn how planning ahead can help you make better decisions.
- Satiety 1
  - Discover the recipe of diet, exercise, and lifestyle change that will elevate your energy expenditure and stop your brain from sending hunger signals.

- Satiety 2
  - ○ Effectively control your metabolism and hunger by consuming certain foods in your diet.
- Self-Monitoring for Success
  - ○ Meal tracking is the key to successful weight loss and maintenance. We'll help you to learn how to consistently track your meals, managing portion size and overcoming the many obstacles that could get in your way.
- Sleep 1
  - ○ Sleep-- the easiest solution to improving mental performance, weight loss, and overall health.
- Sleep 2
  - ○ A simple change in your diet can affect your sleep patterns and be your solution to improved sleep.
- Stress 1
  - ○ Discover how stress directly affects weight gain.
- Stress 2
  - ○ Learn about physical, mental, and interpersonal stress responses and how to effectively manage your stressors.
- Stress 3
  - ○ Assess the stress in your life, identify warning signals, and create your own stress-related first aid kit.
- Denial
  - ○ Overcome your denial and feel better about your health.
- Dining Right 1
  - ○ Learn how to manage the variety of challenges you encounter when eating restaurant meals. Enjoy dining out while dining right!

- Dining Right 2
  - Practice mindful eating. Slow down, enjoy your food, and stick with your program.

- Disordered Eating
  - Equip yourself with important information about disordered eating and how these chaotic eating patterns are triggered.

- Fish Oil-The Fountain of Youth
  - Discover the benefits of fish oil, including prevention of high blood pressure and many other conditions.

- Vitamins and Minerals 1
  - What foods are the good sources of Vitamins C, E, and beta carotene, and what are the recommended daily allowances.

- Vitamins and Minerals 2
  - Discover why you need vitamins and minerals such as folic acid, co-enzyme Q10, calcium, and many more. Are supplements like ginseng and ginkgo biloba really beneficial?

- Water Does a Body Good
  - How much water does your body need? Learn how water plays an important role in weight loss.

- Calories Comparison 1
  - Discover how consuming too much sugar affects your body's chemical balance.

- Calories Comparison 2
  - Watch out for beverages, appetizers, and side dishes that offer nothing but empty calories.

- Calories Comparison 3
  - Manage your calorie intake and make good choices even when eating pizza and fast food.

- Carbs and Sugar 1
  - Learn how consuming refined carbohydrates and sugars will keep you on the constant search for food.

- Carbs and Sugar 2
  - Don't be tricked by food manufacturers who mislead consumers by referring to sugar by other names in their food products.

- Carbs and Sugar 3
  - Did you know sweetened beverages disrupt your body's chemical balance and create bad habits?

- Carbs and Sugar 4
  - Discover how sugars and other carbs cause you to crave them even more, especially in the afternoon and evening.

- Reward Center Eating 1
  - Learn how certain foods stimulate your brain's reward center and how to double your chances of maintaining weight loss.

- Reward Center Eating 2
  - Discover how food engineers create foods to arouse your reward center, causing you to overeat.

- Reward Center Eating 3
  - Why do reward-center foods trigger a cue-craving-reward habit? Learn how to break the cycle.

- Reward Center Eating 4
  - Why can't I stop overeating? Learn how to reprogram your brain and replace bad habits with healthy new behaviors.

- Reward Center Eating 5
  - Developing if-then cognitive responses is key when encountering and overcoming reward-center foods.

- Reward Center Eating 6
  - Practice and perfect your if-then cognitive plans. Discover the acronym HALT NOW.
- Good Fats vs. Bad Fats 1
  - Understand the importance of fat in your diet while learning about insulin resistance. Get the scoop on saturated and unsaturated fats.
- Good Fats vs. Bad Fats 2
  - Get your kitchen in shape to help reduce your fat intake. Learn to prepare healthy low-fat meals with helpful cooking and shopping tips.

Additionally, your wellness program should be able to provide information to your management and your employees on OSHA guidelines and regulations. They should also be able to help you provide healthy meals and snacks in company cafeterias and vending machines.

We strongly recommend offering incentive points to encourage employees to view the videos and pass a short quiz on the videos' content.

One of the best forms of helping to educate and encourage your employees to adapt healthy lifestyles is by providing health club memberships to insured employees and families.

A study by the Prudential Insurance Company on 1389 employees found that fitness memberships resulted in a 20% decrease in the participants' disability days and employee absenteeism days. The Canadian Life Insurance Company found that employee turnover was reduced by 13% by providing fitness memberships for their employees. Many other studies also show that investing in health club memberships produces a very positive ROI.

As we have been saying, trying to save money on good healthcare often costs much more in the long run. The same applies to fitness club memberships. It is important to choose a fitness club that:

- Has qualified staff to provide information on healthy living.
- Regularly communicates health tips to its members by way of newsletter or magazine.
- Provides clean and sanitary equipment and locker rooms. This is especially important to control the spread of illness to your employees.
- Provides enough equipment that your employees and insured families don't wind up spending their workout time waiting for equipment that is being used by others.
- Has equipment that is regularly maintained. Broken or poorly maintained equipment can lead to your employees or families being injured.
- Has multiple activities and classes, so all employees or insured family members can find a fitness activity they enjoy.
- Provides safe childcare so all insured family members can participate.

As with all healthcare providers, it is essential that you be very selective in your choice of a fitness club.

# MANAGING MANDATORY PREVENTIVE CARE

As we discussed in Chapter One, the Affordable Healthcare Act (ACA) mandates that every insurance plan provide a long list of "preventive" tests and procedures at no cost to the insured. We also listed the costs of these procedures[39], which to say the least, were staggering.

39. Appendix A, contains the complete list of these procedures.

Most of your employees and insured families will not have all of these tests and procedures performed. However, there are some tests, such as mammograms, that the majority of women over 40 do have performed regularly. Clearly, in order to have any chance of controlling your company's medical costs, these "preventive" costs must be managed. Having your insured employees and family members obtain these services on their own, often at multiple providers will obviously lead to much higher medical costs for your company.

The 20/20 LifeStyles Wellness Program contracts with a few select providers to perform the commonly used, mandated services such as mammograms or colonoscopies. These medical services can be performed at the providers' convenient locations, and you can direct your insured employees and families to them. We have found that companies achieve very significant savings using this approach.

As we indicated in the table in Chapter One, hospital-owned medical practices actually cost over twice as much for these services as independent medical practices for many reasons, including the "facility fee" they tack on to every visit. Therefore it is essential to direct your insured employees and families to your contracted providers for their preventive care. The best way to do that is by ensuring the services are delivered in the most convenient and time- efficient way. In other words, no long waits in waiting rooms; convenient locations; rapid turn-around on results, and friendly, competent staff.

## HEALTHY MOM-HEALTHY BABY

In Chapter Four we discussed the enormous costs involved in problem pregnancies and childbirths. We mentioned the average cost for a premature birth is $150,000 but can run much, much higher. Even one or two of these incidents in a fiscal year can have a serious impact on your bottom line. As part of their prevention package, your wellness program must provide a comprehensive, effective pregnancy risk-management program.

It has been shown that almost 25% of women have folic acid levels that are too low for safe childbirth. Simply coaching the expectant mother or the woman considering pregnancy to take proper prenatal vitamins will avoid her having a baby with neurological defects like spina bifida and encephalopathy. Low thyroid in the mother during pregnancy also causes several complications that can easily be avoided by a simple blood test and appropriate thyroid medication if needed.

A woman of normal weight can gain up to 20-to-25 pounds during pregnancy. A woman who is overweight before and/or during pregnancy is much more likely to have an obese baby. Large babies are much more likely to cause delivery problems that result in the mother having a premature delivery or a C-section, causing increased discomfort to the mother and increased cost for the employer. Remember, each day a baby is in the neonatal intensive care unit costs $4,400.

Post-pregnancy insurance coverage for "comprehensive support and counseling" is now required by the Federal Government for breastfeeding women.

This is the 20/20 LifeStyles Pregnancy Management Module:

1. *Pre-pregnancy, healthy baby program:*

    a. Two dietitian visits.

    b. Use of 20/20 LifeStyles online meal tracker plus dietitian review.

    c. Two visits with exercise physiologist.

    d. Problem pregnancy costs the company: $150,000+

    e. Program cost $625.

    f. ROI breakeven: immediate.

2. *Pregnancy program:*

    a. Twelve dietitian visits.

    b. Use of 20/20 LifeStyles online meal tracker plus dietitian review.

    c. Four visits with exercise physiologist.

    d. Problem pregnancy costs the company: $150,000+

    e. Program cost $1,220.

    f. ROI breakeven: immediate.

3. *Post-pregnancy program (helps mother return to normal weight and better understand the baby's nutritional needs-this meets federal requirements):*

    a. Two dietitian visits.

    b. One session with exercise physiologist.

    c. Post-pregnancy mother and/or baby health issues costs the company: Can be very high (unknown amount). If mother fails to lose the weight gained during pregnancy, she can develop metabolic disorders like type 2 diabetes, high blood pressure or high cholesterol which will need long term medical treatment.

    d. Program cost $220

    e. ROI breakeven: immediate.

# REPETITIVE STRESS INJURY PREVENTION

OSHA has estimated that 33% of all workmen's compensation dollars are spent on repetitive stress injuries. It is estimated that repetitive stress injuries cost companies in the United States over $20 billion per year. Regardless of employees' jobs, they are at risk for repetitive stress injuries. This is the 20/20 LifeStyles Repetitive Stress Injury Prevention Program:

*Employer onsite ergonomics management module-preventive care program:*

  a. On-site physical therapy evaluation.
  b. Physical therapy report to employer.
  c. Repetitive stress injury (RSI) costs to the company: About $60,000[40].
  d. Program cost $250.
  e. ROI breakeven: immediate.

# EMPLOYEE ADVOCACY—CASE MANAGEMENT MODULE

In order to keep your healthcare costs controllable, it is essential that you are able to manage the medical treatment of your employees and their families. As we have mentioned before, the most cost-effective healthcare is the best healthcare. However, average healthcare consumers find that it is almost impossible to navigate the healthcare system and get their needs met. They may have multiple questions, like:

• How can you find the best doctor for your condition?
• How do you know which medication is best?
• Should you have surgery or try non-surgical treatment?
• How can you contact your doctor on Saturday night when you are feeling ill?

---

40. *For carpal tunnel syndrome. $30,000 in workers' compensation and $33,000 in indirect medical costs. Source OSHA cost estimator.*

Without assistance, these issues and many other confusing medical questions will not be resolved effectively with the best treatment for the employee and the lowest overall cost for the company.

When employees or their families are confused and/or anxious, they often wind up in the emergency room of the local hospital. The CDC reports that 79.7% of emergency room admissions were due to the patients' "lack of access to other providers[41]." The average cost of a visit to a family physician ranges from $60 to $175. The average cost of visits to the emergency room is **$3400**. 20/20 LifeStyles provides case management and physician availability to answer medical questions. THIS IS NOT "MANAGED CARE."

Health care consumers hate managed care, and managed care does not save money. The 20/20 LifeStyles doctors earn the trust of the employees they work with. They are not the cold voice on the phone talking to them from another state or country. The employees have met and talked to these doctors, and they have seen that the program doctors have the employee's best interest as their goal. Our doctors cut through the red tape, confusion, and delay and get the employees treated promptly and by the best medical professionals. They follow up with the employees to be sure they have everything they need and their questions are answered. Our doctors then continue to ensure the employees receive the most effective treatment and continue meeting with the employees and coordinating their care until their medical issues are resolved or stable.

As an option, the 20/20 LifeStyles doctors also are available to see employees for "sick call" at one of their locations or at on-site locations in your company's facilities. Using this "sick call" our doctors can treat most medical problems immediately with no employee time loss. The problems they can't treat on-site are referred to a pre-screened group of medical providers, assuring the most effective treatment.

41. *Emergency Room Use Among Adults, Gindi, et. Al. ,CDC, May 2012.*

20/20 LifeStyles case management is a win-win situation. The company saves money because treatment is efficiently provided by the best medical providers, and the employees feel a strong loyalty to the company for the help they received.

So I ask you, does your wellness program do this for you?

# CHAPTER 9

## 20/20 LIFESTYLES
## TREATMENT MODULES-PART 1

---

## WOUND PRETTY TIGHT

### CHARLEY - Group Manager for a Technology Company

I was a group manager for a local technology company, and I was one of their top performers. My team always produced results, no matter how difficult the project or how short the timeline, and my company rewarded me well for that. I had a great house in a beautiful part of town, I loved my wife, and I had two kids doing great in college. I was living the American dream.

But one Friday reality came crashing down on me when I had a mid-year review with my V.P. He told me that the turnover rate in my group was five times normal compared to his other groups and that several of my peers had complained about my being very intense and demanding. He said that if things didn't change I wouldn't be getting a good year-end review. I told him I would work on it, but I didn't have a clue what he was talking about. I pressed hard, but how else could I get the results I had achieved?

When I got home that night my wife immediately knew that something was wrong. I told her about my meeting with the V.P., and she was strangely quiet. When I asked what was wrong she said, "I agree with your V.P., stress seems to follow you around." Well, that absolutely floored me. I didn't know what to feel or say.

I didn't sleep much that night and when I went to work the next day I was still depressed and confused.

At that time, my company was making a big push to get people signed up for their new 20/20 LifeStyles Wellness program. As a group manager, I felt I had to set a good example for my team, so I decided to attend one of their lectures. Talk about a life-changing decision!

The 20/20 LifeStyles psychologist was giving a brown bag lunch talk that day, so I went. His topic for that talk was stress and its effects. At first I barely listened as I thought about everything I had to do that day. But as he went on, a bomb exploded in my brain. HE WAS TALKING ABOUT ME!

He told us that stress caused the body to overproduce cortisol and that cortisol caused you to gain weight and develop a long list of metabolic problems. But worse yet, he said stress is contagious. He said research had shown that when a stressed individual interacts with others, within 15 minutes the others have elevated stress levels. All of a sudden I realized that was me, "typhoid Charley." I realized that I was driving my workgroup and my wife crazy.

I signed up with the 20/20 LifeStyles Wellness Program that same day. Two days later I filled out the online lifestyles questionnaire and had my biometric testing and blood draw. The following Monday I met with the 20/20 LifeStyles doctor and got my results. As you can guess, the news was not good.

I was 40 pounds overweight, had high blood pressure, high cholesterol, and was pre-diabetic. He said that he was quite concerned that at 47 years of age I had already developed three metabolic disorders and was progressing toward a fourth.

I told him about the brown bag lunch on stress that I had attended and that I thought stress was the root of my medical problems. He totally agreed. He told me he could prescribe medications for my blood pressure and cholesterol and refer me to a psychiatrist to prescribe medication for my stress. He also said that in his experience medications didn't seem to help very much with stress, and he strongly recommended that I sign up for 20/20 LifeStyles Stress Program, which was covered by my company.

Well, I didn't like the news, but the doctor impressed me with his knowledge and honesty, so I signed up.

Because of what I learned from 20/20 LifeStyles, I never took one drug for my stress or metabolic disorders. Not one. I lost the 40 pounds, corrected my cholesterol and high blood pressure, and I also regained my energy and endurance. But best of all, the lifestyle counseling, learning good nutrition, and developing healthy exercise habits eliminated the stress that was destroying my life and the life of everyone around me. Everyone around me has commented on how much more relaxed I am, and my wife even wrote a thank you note to 20/20 LifeStyles.

I know that sounds impossible to some people, but I'm living proof.

If I can leave you with one thought, it's this: Health is a matter of choice. You have it in your power to choose the right lifestyle and the right state of mind. You have the final responsibility for your health. If you haven't taken responsibility for your health and life yet, I encourage you to be like me and do it. Not tomorrow but today.

# STRESS AND DEPRESSION IN THE WORKPLACE

Charley's stress caused his health problems. It also caused problems for his company due to the high turnover rate in Charley's group and the stress that everyone who worked with Charley "caught" from him.

Forty percent (40%) of all job turnover is due to stress. Healthcare expenditures are 50% higher for employees who are feeling stress. Claims for industrial injuries of employees reporting stress are double those of employees not reporting stress[42].

Each year about 10% of the population will suffer clinical depression. In a 90-day period depressed employees miss an average of five workdays plus 12 days of decreased productivity [43].

Stress and depression account for 46% of all work absences. Also, the presenteeism caused by stress and depression costs twice as much as the total cost of all absenteeism[44]. So let's see why that happens.

When you have physical stress, emotional stress, or depression, your body undergoes many chemical changes. These changes were designed to help your hunter-gatherer ancestors survive a crisis situation. They're called fight-or-flight responses.

One of those changes happens when the adrenal gland, a small gland on top of the kidney, contracts to cause increased secretion of three substances. Two of these chemicals, norepinephrine and epinephrine, make you more mentally agile and heighten your awareness. The third chemical is cortisol, a corticosteroid.

42. *University of Massachusetts, Stress@Work.*
43. *CDC Workplace Health Promotion.*
44. *Journal of Occupational Medicine.*

Many of you have heard of the medications cortisone, prednisone, or prednisolone. All these also belong to a class called corticosteroids. Some of you may have even had these medications prescribed to reduce inflammation related to a medical condition. Many patients who take corticosteroids have significant and rapid weight gains. If you suffer from stress, depression, or both, your body produces an excess of these corticosteroids.

As for stress, one can have either acute or chronic stress.

In prehistoric times, when our ancestors who were gathering nuts and berries came across a saber-tooth tiger, they experienced acute stress. Luckily, our ancestors' bodies had this built-in fight-or-flight chemical change that allowed them to think fast and run fast. If that ancestor was frightened or, worse, injured, a cortisol burst helped him to function well enough to avoid becoming disabled and tiger food. One way or the other, his acute stress resolved in a relatively short time.

Chronic stress and depression are, however, long-term conditions. They can be caused by physical illness or injury but are more often due to long-standing life and emotional problems. If your problems are financial, work, family, or relationship issues, they can be persistent challenges you deal with all day, every day. In response, your body may constantly be producing an overabundance of norepinephrine, epinephrine, and cortisol. As we've pointed out, excess cortisol can make you gain weight, and worse yet, it can cause insulin resistance, moving you into the cycle of high cholesterol, high blood pressure, weight gain, and, eventually, type 2 diabetes (Figure 1).

*Figure 1*

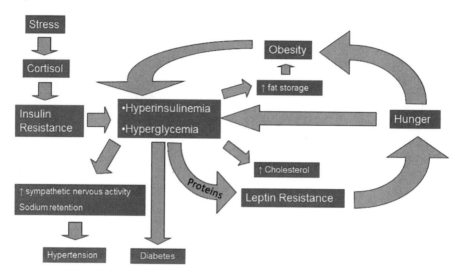

As you can see, the cortisol released in response to stress (and depression) has triggered a cascade of events. The result is a metabolic disaster, caused by insulin resistance.

Stress and depression can cause:

- Heart disease
- Cancer
- Gastrointestinal problems
- Infections
- Arthritis
- High cholesterol
- High blood pressure
- Type 2 diabetes
- Asthma
- Headaches
- Fatigue
- Weight gain
- Suppression of the immune system

We've described how we work with a company's management team and with their employees, and you've seen examples of how the 20/20 LifeStyles Wellness Program works with some typical employee health issues. Now we will address specific treatment programs for employees with chronic illnesses or risk factors for chronic illness. You will notice that as we present these modules we will also discuss program costs and ROI, because we believe it is essential for a wellness program to always be able to show a positive ROI. 20/20 LifeStyles shows costs and return on investment for all of its Wellness Program Modules.

# STRESS AND DEPRESSION MODULES

We've discussed how stress and depression not only cause your healthcare costs to increase dramatically but also cost you three times that amount in presenteeism, absenteeism, worker's compensation, and disability costs. Remember stress is responsible for 13% of all absences. Employee stress can range from the mild stress of a home remodel to the severe stress of a family disruption due to divorce, illness, or work problems.

Stressed employees cost you money! The direct and indirect medical costs for stressed employees are:

- Mild stress - $1,900 per year

- Moderate stress - $3700 per year

- Severe Stress - $6900 per year

Stress management is a vital part of a successful wellness program, yet many wellness programs either ignore it or offer minimal services to deal with it. 20/20 LifeStyles has stress management modules for different levels of stress. This is the 20/20 LifeStyles Stress Management Module:

1. *Mild stress management program:*
   a. Three stress management videos viewed online.
   b. Two visits with psychologist.
   c. Mild stress costs the company: $1,900 per year.
   d. Program cost $285.
   e. ROI break even: two months.

2. *Moderate stress management program:*
   a. Three stress videos viewed online.
   b. Twelve visits with psychologist.
   c. Medication evaluation.
   d. Two dietitian visits.
   e. Two exercise physiologist sessions.
   f. Moderate stress costs the company: $3,700 per year.
   g. Program cost $2,035.
   h. ROI break even: seven months.

3. *Severe stress management program:*
   a. Three stress videos viewed online.
   b. Twenty-four visits with psychologist.
   c. Medication evaluation plus medication follow-up visit.
   d. Two dietitian visits.
   e. Two exercise physiologist sessions.
   f. Severe stress costs the company: $6,900 per year.
   g. Program cost $4,125.
   h. ROI break even: seven months.

Almost everyone has depression at some point in their lives, and depression is not only very unpleasant, it is also disabling. Additionally, as we mentioned before, depression leads to several serious medical illnesses. It also is a major cause of presenteeism and absenteeism. Furthermore it is one of the leading causes of short-term and long-term disability. The direct and indirect medical costs for depressed employees are:

- Mild depression - $3,700 per year
- Moderate depression - $5,800 per year
- Severe depression - $15,000 per year (but can be much higher)

This is the 20/20 LifeStyles Depression Management Module:

1. Mild depression management program:
   a. Three stress videos viewed online.
   b. Two depression videos viewed online.
   c. Six visits with psychologist.
   d. Mild depression costs the company: $3,700 per year.
   e. Program cost $835
   f. ROI break even: three months.

2. Moderate depression management program:
   a. Three stress videos viewed online.
   b. Two depression videos viewed online
   c. Twelve in-person visits with psychologist.
   d. Four dietitian visits.
   e. Eight sessions with exercise physiologist.
   f. Moderate depression costs the company: $5,800 per year.
   g. Program cost $2,685.
   h. ROI break even: 5.5 months.

In severe depression, the depressed individual will have already been placed on an antidepressant medication by his family physician. Frequently that individual is unable to work and is receiving disability pay. And frequently these people are hospitalized at a cost of $2,000 per day. This is the 20/20 LifeStyles severe Depression Management Module:

3. *Severe depression management program:*
   a. Twenty-two visits with psychologist.
   b. Dietitian visits weekly for 12 weeks and every other week for 12 weeks.

c. Exercise physiologist visits three days per week for 12 weeks and twice per week for 12 weeks.

d. 60 videos to watch while warming up for workouts.

e. 20/20 LifeStyles online tracker to Track food, monitored by dietitian.

f. Medication evaluation plus medication follow-up visit.

g. Severe depression costs the company: $15,000 per year and can be much more if hospitalization is required.

h. Program cost $12,105.

i. ROI breakeven: 10 months.

Financial problems often lead to long-term stress and depression. Employees with severe financial problems often lose productivity, find it difficult to concentrate, and become angry and irritable. They may try to find second jobs, which cause them to be extremely fatigued at work and prone to mistakes and injuries.

This is the 20/20 LifeStyles Financial Health Management Module:

*Financial Health management program.*

a. Three stress videos viewed online.

b. Two depression videos viewed online.

c. Three visits with psychologist.

d. Three visits with financial counselor

e. Severe stress related to finances costs the company: $6,900 per year.

f. Program cost $835

g. ROI breakeven: 1.5 months.

# SLEEP DISORDER MODULE

Unfortunately in today's fast-paced, high-stress world, we often deprive ourselves of sleep in order to accommodate our overscheduled lifestyle. In fact over the last 40 years Americans have decreased their nightly sleep by almost 25%. Where we used to sleep for 8½ hours, we now sleep for six or seven.

"About 70 million Americans suffer from chronic sleep problems. Employees with sleep disorders are often problem employees. Inadequate or insufficient sleep is associated with injuries, chronic diseases, mental illnesses, poor quality of life and well-being, increased health care costs, and lost work productivity. Sleep problems are critically under-addressed contributors to some chronic conditions, including obesity and depression[45]."

Sleep apnea is a condition that causes an individual to stop breathing frequently while sleeping. The result is that the person is unable to get deep, restorative sleep. Sleep apnea causes chronic sleep deprivation, which reduces brain function and damages the body. This sleep deficit is associated with stroke, weight gain, cardiovascular disease, diabetes, industrial injury, motor vehicle accident[46], high blood pressure, attention deficit disorder, and problem pregnancies and births.

In the 20/20 LifeStyles Program we have found that most very obese individuals have sleep apnea and that sleep disorders are very strongly related to weight gain, which in turn causes the cascade of metabolic disorders listed above. The direct and indirect medical cost for sleep deprived employees is $2900 to $4,200 per year. This is the 20/20 LifeStyles Sleep Management Module:

45. CDC, July 2013.
46. NHTSA estimates sleep disorder responsible for 100,000 accidents per year.

1. *Mild to moderate sleep management program:*
    a. View two sleep videos online.
    b. Attend sleep workshop at employer facility.
    c. Visit with psychologist.
    d. Visit with dietitian.
    e. Visit with exercise physiologist.
    f. Mild to moderate sleep disorders costs the company: $2,900 per year.
    g. Program cost $330.
    h. ROI breakeven: 1.4 months.

2. Moderate to severe sleep management program:
    a. View two sleep videos online.
    b. Attend sleep workshop at employer facility.
    c. Visit with psychologist.
    d. Visit with dietitian.
    e. Visit with exercise physiologist.
    f. Have an at-home, overnight sleep-apnea screening.*
    g. Visit with physician specializing in sleep disorders.
    h. Severe sleep disorders costs the company: $4,200 per year.
    i. Program cost $930.
    j. ROI breakeven: 1.1 months.

   *Note: if sleep apnea screening is positive, a full sleep study must be performed. This will increase cost by $1,800 and increase ROI breakeven to 8 months.*

# NECK AND BACK PAIN/REPETITIVE STRESS INJURY MODULE

Neck and low back pain affect 80% of the population of the U.S. at some point in their lives [47]. It is the fifth most common reason for individuals to seek medical treatment. It is second only to upper

47. Freburger, et. al., *Archives of internal Medicine, 2009.*

respiratory infections in days absent from work and accounts for more than 50% of the entire cost of industrial injuries[48].

And, as we mentioned before, 33% of all workmen's compensation dollars are spent on repetitive stress injuries.

20/20 LifeStyles has found that back surgery is warranted less than 5% of the time when an individual presents with back or neck pain. About 95% of back and neck pain can be treated with conservative care, followed by Pilates or other core muscle strengthening techniques.

The direct and indirect medical costs for employees with current neck or low back pain is $3,200 to $4,900 per incident. Obviously this cost can escalate dramatically if the employee requires medical tests such as an MRI or procedures such as steroid injections and surgery. This is the 20/20 LifeStyles Neck and Low Back Pain/Repetitive Stress Injury Management Module:

1. *Mild to moderate Neck and low back pain/repetitive stress injury management program:*
   a. Initial visit and follow-up with 20/20 LifeStyles orthopedic physician.
   b. X-rays if necessary.
   c. Visit with specific pressure point massage therapist.*
   d. Four visits to physical therapist.
   e. Four sessions with exercise physiologist certified in Pilates body alignment, flexibility, and strengthening.
   f. Mild to moderate neck or back pain costs the company: $3,200 per year.
   g. Program cost $1,250
   h. ROI breakeven: five months.**

   *This often corrects the problem, and no further treatment is needed.*
   **If treatment avoids one back surgery for every 25 visits the ROI is immediate.*

48. *University of Missouri, School of Health Professions.*

2. *Moderate to severe Neck and low back pain/repetitive stress injury management program:*
   a. Initial visit and follow up with 20/20 LifeStyles orthopedic physician.
   b. An MRI.
   c. Four visits to physical therapist.
   d. Four sessions with exercise physiologist certified in Pilates body alignment, flexibility, and strengthening.
   e. Three visits to orthopedic physician for injection therapy.
   f. Moderate to severe neck or back pain costs the company: $4,900 per year.
   g. Program cost $2,700.
   h. ROI breakeven: seven months.*

   *If treatment avoids one back surgery for every 15 visits the ROI is immediate.*

# CHAPTER 10

## 20/20 LIFESTYLES
## TREATMENT MODULES-PART 2

---

### A BIG GUY
*Sean - Partner in a Large Law Firm*

I was always a big guy. I even played a little college ball. I was 6-foot-1, weighed in at 248 and was in great shape. When I got my law degree, I got hired by a good-sized firm for a great salary.

That's when I really learned what hard work was all about. Being a new guy in a law firm meant working about 70 hours a week. My job became my whole life. I slept about five hours a night, skipped breakfast, and ate lunch and dinner at the office. I ran on caffeine and sugar. If I got a day off on a weekend, I'd watch football, drink beer, and eat chips and pizza.

I would brag that my weight hadn't changed since college, but the fact is my waist size had gone up considerably. Muscle is a lot more compact than fat!

I turned 46 and decided to have the physical, which I'd been avoiding. I was really shocked. My doctor was a good guy and had been our family doctor for many years, so I trusted and respected him. He sat me down and said that I was in real trouble. My blood pressure was up, my cholesterol was up, and my blood sugar was up. He said that I was a type 2 diabetic and a heart attack waiting to happen. Then he prescribed a bunch of medications for me and told me to come back in a month.

I was pretty shook up.

We had a wellness program at work for several years, and a couple of years ago I had attended a couple of "brown bag lunches" given by one of their people. They seemed competent and seemed to know what they were talking about, but I really didn't ever have the time to get involved with the program. I did remember one thing they said: that medication only treats the symptom, but lifestyle change treats the disease.

I called the 20/20 LifeStyles Wellness Program and talked to one of their intake people. I explained my situation to her and she told me that 20/20 LifeStyles could correct my problem without medication.

She scheduled me to attend a 2½-hour introductory seminar. I'm a very busy guy and really didn't want to waste an evening listening to some lecture, but this one was really different. It was delivered by no less than a cardiovascular surgeon, and what he said convinced me of two things: He really knew what he was talking about and I was in big trouble with my health. Well, I signed up for the program and when I got home that evening, they had already emailed me instructions to complete my online health and lifestyle questionnaire.

Much to my surprise the first person I met with was a psychologist. I asked why I was meeting with a psychologist. I really didn't think I was crazy, but then I suspect most people who are crazy don't think so either. He explained to me that my medical problems were caused by my lifestyle and he was the lifestyle expert. He did a complete assessment of my history, including work history, diet history, and fitness history. He also explained a bit about the program and told me that clients who had been former athletes usually did exceptionally well in the program. He explained that my next stop would be to have blood drawn, then measurements in the performance lab and a meeting with the medical doctor. I'll tell you, I left that office feeling pretty darn good. This wasn't a "one size fits all" type of program; they really wanted to know about me.

In the performance lab they took several measurements of my body, tested my strength, flexibility and gave me my percent body fat and muscle. This gave them a complete understanding of my overall health, cardiovascular fitness, and overall fitness level.

I also had my personal doctor fax them my medical records. All of this information had been sent to the program doctor and when I met with him, I found that he had read it all and knew my history. He spent an hour with me reviewing my test data, gave me a copy of it (about 15 pages), and then gave me a comprehensive lifestyle prescription. It covered everything: my nutrition plan, exercise plan and my limitations, what vitamins I should take, and how many hours of sleep I needed. He also told me that he had calculated my physiological age to be 58. Not too good for a 47 year old.

Next I met with my dietitian. She explained the nutrition portion of the program and taught me how to use the 20/20 LifeStyles online meal tracker and online tools. She had a pretty slick set-up with one computer screen facing her and one facing me, so she could take me through everything I needed to know. She informed me that when I entered my food in my meal tracker, she would be able to review it on her computer. She then set me up on Stage 1 of the program's food plan and told me we would be meeting weekly. Finally she told me to email, text, or call with any questions and she would get right back to me.

My last stop was with my personal trainer, and I need to tell you I was a bit nervous about this one. In college my training sessions had been really demanding, and I knew trying to be that ambitious now would probably kill me. But to my surprise, before I even stepped on a treadmill, my trainer reviewed the complete performance lab assessment of my physical abilities and explained how we would work. Before I worked out, I would warm up on a recumbent bike with a video screen built in to it. There were 60 educational videos that I would watch during the program, so that I could learn how my body functioned and how my lifestyle, behaviors, and habits had caused me to gain weight and develop my metabolic disorders.

You know, I'm not easy to impress, but I was really impressed. These guys were the gold standard. I was really pumped and ready to get started.

I was in the program for a total of seven months including the 12 week aftercare. I had my blood tests, measurements and doctor visits two more times.

I lost 68 pounds and was at a normal weight of 180 pounds, my blood pressure, cholesterol and blood sugar was normal. Best of all my physiologic age was down to 32. All this without ever having to take any medications.

As if the fact that our corporate wellness program saved my life weren't enough, here's the rest of the story. My wife and kids are much healthier now. And, instead of being couch potatoes, we eat right, hike, bike, and ski together.

My work output has really increased, I'm able to accomplish more work faster, and I have landed an impressive list of clients. One of our managing partners is retiring next year, I feel like I have a good shot at that position. You know, life is really good.

# OVERWEIGHT AND METABOLIC DISORDER MODULE

Individuals who are overweight or obese have a significantly increased chance of developing the following medical conditions:

- Type 2 diabetes.
- High blood pressure.

- High cholesterol and triglycerides.
- Coronary artery disease and heart attack.
- Stroke.
- Cancer-colon, breast, ovarian, kidney, esophagus, stomach, pancreas, and prostate.
- Gall stones.
- Gout.
- Sleep apnea.
- Fatty liver disease.
- Infertility.
- Asthma.
- Osteoarthritis.
- Back, muscle, and joint pain.

Overweight and obese employees miss **450 MILLION** more days of work each year than their normally weighted coworkers, which costs business $153 billion dollars in lost productivity due to absenteeism. They cost 42% more in direct medical expenses on an annual basis. They also filed twice the number of worker's compensation claims, had seven times higher cost per claim, and lost an average of 13 days more per claim than normally weighted employees[49]. Finally, obese and overweight employees suffered a 4.2% presenteeism penalty (they produced 4.2% less than normally weighted workers). As startling as these statistics are, they don't even begin to address the corporate cost of the diseases listed above.

The 20/20 LifeStyles Overweight and Metabolic Disorder treatment module has proven successful for over 20 years, for more than 10,000 participants. During these years the module has been continually improved using state-of-the-art medical science. Today 20/20 LifeStyles is the most successful non-surgical weight loss and metabolic disease program in the world.

49. *Archives of Internal Medicine, April 23, 2007.*

The success of 20/20 LifeStyles can be seen in the chart below. The remission rates listed in this chart indicate that the program participant discontinued all medications for the condition, had normal biometrics, and no longer had any symptoms of the disorder. Those remission rates are very impressive, but they still don't tell the whole story.

The table below shows the annual costs for and individual with one of the most common metabolic disorders as well as the 20/20 LifeStyles complete remission rates for those disorders:

| Condition or Disorder | Annual Direct & Indirect Medical Cost | 20/20 LifeStyles Remission Rate |
|---|---|---|
| High Cholesterol | $5,400 | 79% |
| High Blood Pressure | $4,100 | 61% |
| Type 2 Diabetes | $13,700 | 73% |
| Depression | $5,800 | 68% |
| Fibromyalgia | $7,100 | 85% |
| Osteoarthritis | $8,000 | 86% |
| Obesity | $5,300 | 93% |
| Super Morbid Obesity | $9,400 | 70% |

In addition to those participants who are in complete remission, many of the other participants are in partial remission. That means they have reduced their medication needs significantly, meaning lower dosages and fewer medications (often down from several medications to one or two). Even type 1 diabetics can reduce their insulin needs and more easily control their blood sugars, reducing disabling and costly complications.

The 20/20 LifeStyles Overweight and Metabolic Disorder module is designed to treat overweight and the expensive metabolic disorders that occur as individuals gain weight. Our treatment module begins with a program for individuals who are overweight but have not yet developed the associated metabolic disorders.

Note that ROI break-even points are calculated based on company savings in medications and other healthcare expenses as well as reduction or elimination of indirect medical costs. The direct and indirect corporate medical costs for overweight and obese employees are:

- Uncomplicated overweight (BMI 27-30) - $5,300 per year
- Overweight (BMI 27-30) plus at least one risk factor[50] - $9,515
- Obesity (BMI 31-35) plus at least one risk factor - $12,067
- Severe metabolic disorder program (BMI 36-40) plus risk factors - $17,195
- Very Severe metabolic disorder program (BMI 41+) plus risk factors - $23,004

We are able to perform the following modules using Skype or telephone visits, however we find it is preferable to perform these services in-person when possible. This is the 20/20 LifeStyles Overweight and Metabolic Disorder Treatment Module:

1. *Overweight without metabolic disorders program: BMI 27-30:*

   a. Twelve-week program.

   b. In-person or Skype or phone dietitian sessions weekly for 12 weeks.

   c. Three in-person, phone or Skype sessions with exercise physiologist.

   d. Five in-person, phone or Skype sessions with Lifestyle counselor.

   e. Over 60 online videos to watch.

   f. 20/20 LifeStyles online meal tracker to track food.

   g. Overweight without metabolic disorders costs the company: $5,300 per year.

   h. Program cost $1,695.

   i. ROI breakeven: four months.

2. *Overweight with metabolic disorder/obese[51] program: BMI 27-30*

50. *Risk factors like high blood pressure, high cholesterol, type two diabetes, etc.*

*with at least one major risk factor[52]:*
    a. Twelve-week program plus 12-week maintenance program.
    b. Eighteen in-person dietitian visits.
        i. Twelve weekly visits.
        ii. Six every-other-week visits.
    c. Sixty in-person visits with exercise physiologist.
        i. Three visits weekly for 12 weeks.
        ii. Two visits weekly for 12 weeks.
    d. Five in-person visits with Lifestyle counselor.
    e. Ten group workshops.
    f. 60 videos to watch while warming up for workouts.
    g. 20/20 LifeStyles online tracker, monitored by dietitian, to track food.
    h. Overweight with metabolic disorders costs the company: $17,067 per year.
    i. Program cost $8,800.
    j. ROI breakeven: six months.

3. *Obesity with at least one other risk factor program: BMI 31-35:*
    a. Sixteen-week program plus 12-week maintenance program.
    b. Twenty-two in-person dietitian visits.
        i. Sixteen weekly visits.
        ii. Six every-other-week visits.
    c. Seventy-two in-person visits with exercise physiologist.
        i. Three visits weekly for 16 weeks.
        ii. Two visits weekly for 12 weeks.
    d. Six in-person visits with Lifestyle counselor.
    e. Ten group workshops.
    f. 60 videos to watch while warming up for workouts.

---

51. *Due to repeated attempts at weight loss, individuals may have a very high percentage of body fat and be obese even at a BMI of 27-30.*
52. *Risk factors like high blood pressure, high cholesterol, type two diabetes, etc.*

g. 20/20 LifeStyles online tracker, monitored by dietitian, to track food.

h. Obesity costs the company: $18,500 per year.

i. Program cost $10,290.

j. ROI breakeven: 5.5 months.

*Note that the program length increases as the BMI increases.*

4. *Severe Obesity program: BMI 36-40:*

a. Twenty-week program

b. 12-week maintenance program.

c. Severe obesity costs the company: $20,195 per year

d. Program cost $11,500

e. ROI breakeven: seven months.

5. *Morbid obesity program: BMI 41+:*

a. Twenty-four week program.

b. 12-week maintenance program.

c. Morbid obesity costs the company: $27,004 per year

d. Program cost $12,860

e. ROI breakeven: six months.

We have successfully treated individuals with BMIs as high as 67 weighing 595 pounds. The program cost was $17,400, but the ROI was only three months! The alternative to the 20/20 LifeStyles program for this individual was bariatric surgery. Insurance cost for bariatric surgery is about $30,000, but when you add follow-up visits and complications, the total cost is about $60,000. That doesn't count time absent from work or presenteeism encountered due to complications and permanent side effects of the surgery. Plus a high percentage of individuals undergoing bariatric surgery gain a substantial portion of their weight back in three years. 20/20 LifeStyles has treated over 200 individuals who have had the surgery and then gained all their weight back (usually with additional weight gain).

Because long-term weight maintenance is difficult, we recommend a three-year follow-up program for our participants. The lifestyle habits our participants learn during the 20/20 LifeStyles program are new habits. When people are under stress they often revert to older, more familiar habits, and that means weight gain. We have found that accountability is essential in avoiding relapse and enabling long-term weight maintenance. Having contact (and accountability) with our dietitians for three years helps the individuals continue to focus on their health and weight. At the end of three years their healthy lifestyle habits have become the "old habits" and cannot be easily disrupted.

*Three-year maintenance program:*

1. Seventy-two in-person dietitian visits--two visits per month.

2. On-line weekly dietitian review application.

3. On-line meal tracking at least three days per week.
    a. On-line meal tracking five days per week if three pound weight gain.
    b. On-line meal tracking daily if five pound weight gain.

4. On-line tracking of exercise three days per week.

5. Lifestyle counselor visits if needed.

6. Program cost $780 per year.

7. ROI breakeven immediate.

We strongly recommend motivating employees by giving incentive points for:

• Participating in the needed module.
• Successfully completing a needed module.
• Maintaining long-term weight loss

Employees of companies that use incentive points for achievement have better long-term success rates.

# CHAPTER 11

## 20/20 LIFESTYLES
## TREATMENT MODULES-PART 3

---

## A BAD HABIT

*Jen - Assistant Store Manager for a Retail Company*

I was 32 years old, with an 18-month-old son, and was an assistant store manager for a retail firm. My marriage was great, my son was a joy, I was still in my high school dress size, and I was moving up in my company. Life was really good.

When the flu season hit, my 18-month-old caught it. It was a really nasty flu, and he kept us up for about 10 nights. Sure enough, just as he was getting better, I got sick. The flu hit me really hard, and I was out of work for over a week. My store manager really didn't appreciate it because she had to do her job and mine too.

Our company had started another wellness program, and as part of the management team I was expected to set an example. So, I filled out the health and lifestyles questionnaire and had my biometrics done.

When I met with the 20/20 LifeStyles Wellness Program doctor to discuss the results, he said they were all fine. Then he asked me about my cough. I told him I had the flu awhile ago and had not gotten over it yet. He asked me how long it had been since I had the flu, and I said about six weeks ago. Then he said he noticed from my lifestyles questionnaire that I smoked.

Like all smokers I was concerned about that bad habit, and when he mentioned smoking I got scared.

Because of my persistent cough, he scheduled me for a chest x-ray the next day. He said he wanted to meet with me the day after to discuss the results. Well, that was two anxious days!

When I met with him, he immediately told me my x-ray did not show signs of lung cancer but quickly stated that didn't get me off the hook. The x-ray did show changes in my lungs, and he said the coughing could be related to chronic bronchitis due to my smoking. He said I had two choices: he could schedule me with a lung doctor for a series of tests and then I might have to use an inhaler for the rest of my life, or I could sign up for the 20/20 LifeStyles Smoking Cessation program.

I liked and trusted this doctor, so I told him that I knew smoking is bad for me and I've tried to quit several times. I even managed to stay quit for 9 months during my pregnancy, but I went right back to it after I had my baby. Since my son was born, I haven't even been able to make it a day without a cigarette.

He told me that their smoking cessation program was very intensive and I might really be surprised by the results. Like I said, I trusted him, so I signed up.

I was pleasantly surprised that the first person I met with in the smoking cessation program was a 20/20 LifeStyles nurse practitioner that specialized in smoking cessation. She took a very thorough history of my smoking and overall lifestyle and told me that because I had been able to quit while I was pregnant, that she would start me on a moderate level program. She made it very clear that if I was not initially successful at quitting, I could move up to a higher level.

I was amazed to see that the program she prescribed was a one-year program. She gave me a prescription for Chantix to help with the withdrawal but told me if that didn't work or if I had problems with it, there were a number of other medications she could try.

During that year I attended 3 smoking cessation workshops, had 9 more in-person appointments with the nurse practitioner, as well as 10 video conference calls with her. I won't tell you it was easy because it wasn't. I had a couple of relapses in the first 60 days, and we had to change my medication one time. But I hung in there and did it.

I have been a non-smoker now for three years and I hope my example will mean that my children (now two of them) will follow that example and never smoke. Amazingly without my frequent smoke breaks I was able to accomplish much more at my store and was recently promoted to brand manager at the corporate headquarters. After a couple of months, I lost my smokers cough and you know what, I almost never get the flu or colds anymore. I thought my life was good then, but it's a lot better now.

## SMOKING CESSATION MODULE

In Chapter Seven we discussed the corporate costs of employees who smoke. We stated that smokers cost their company $5,300 dollars per year[53][54]. This includes only the cost of direct medical care. It does NOT include the costs for absenteeism (6.16 days per year) and presenteeism which accounts for a reduction of over 8% in productivity (a loss of one month's productivity per year due to time spent on smoke breaks). Also, it does not take into account the very serious and costly illnesses like lung cancer, heart disease, and emphysema caused by smoking.

Jen's smoking cessation program cost her company $2,950. For ROI purposes this is only compared to the $10,000 a year for direct and indirect medical costs.

53. *These are medical costs for colds, sinus infections, headaches, influenza, and pneumonia, which smokers are much more likely to contract.*
54. *National Business Group on Health*

In Jen's case, however, the costs were going to be much higher. Her testing would have consisted of a full pulmonary function study, a high resolution CT scan of the chest, and at least two visits with a pulmonologist. Total cost close to $4,000. Next she might have been placed on an inhaler, which would be an on-going cost. And she would continue to have severe colds and influenza, which would also run up her medical bills. Lastly her smoking would have caused her to develop a serious disease like emphysema, heart disease, or cancer. The ROI on Jen's smoking cessation program was 9 months. Not only that but she has become a much more valuable employee and has set an example of hope for her "smoking group."

Taking a closer look at Jen's program, the first thing that you notice is that it is a long- term intensive treatment program. The reason for that is because smoking addiction is extremely resistant to current treatment modalities. Statistics for long-term, successful treatment outcomes are not very good. Standard care with medications and lectures yields a success rate of about 10.9% after one year. Models using engaged care, where the smoker has regular meetings with a "quit smoking counselor," do a bit better at 13.5%. The 20/20 LifeStyles Program has a 28.5% success rate after one year.

We feel that the results generated by state of the art treatment modalities are not very good, and we are continually trying to improve our model. However, as it stands today we still have results that are twice as good as the other programs.

This is the 20/20 LifeStyles Smoking Cessation Module:

1. *One year mild dependence treatment program:*
    a. Initial medical assessment.
    b. Two group workshops.
    c. Six online Skype sessions with psychologist.
    d. Six visits with psychologist.

    e. Smoking costs the company: about $10,000 per year.

    f. Program cost $1,450.

    g. ROI breakeven: 2 months.

2. One year moderate dependence treatment program"

    a. Initial medical assessment.

    b. Three group workshops.

    c. Ten online Skype sessions with nurse practitioner.

    d. Nine sessions with nurse practitioner.

    e. Medication for smoking cessation.

    f. Smoking costs the company: about $10,000 per year.

    g. Program cost $2,950.

    h. ROI breakeven: 3.5 months.

3. One year severe dependence treatment program:

    a. Initial medical assessment.

    b. Four group workshops.

    c. Fourteen online Skype sessions with nurse practitioner.

    d. Twelve sessions with nurse practitioner.

    e. Medication for smoking cessation (combination of medications).

    f. Smoking costs the company: about $10,000 per year.

    g. Program cost $4,500.

    h. ROI breakeven: 5 months.

# CHAPTER 12

## 20/20 LIFESTYLES
## TREATMENT MODULES-PART 4

---

## MONDAY, BLOODY MONDAY
*Cindy - Assembly Line Worker for a Manufacturing Company*

I worked for a company that did light manufacturing, and I worked on the assembly line. I was 28 years old, divorced, and had a 10-year-old daughter. I didn't really like my job, but it was pretty easy and I had to support my daughter and myself. I'd worked for the company for five years, which is probably the reason they didn't fire me.

I felt I had a hard life. After all, I was a 28-year-old single mom working on an assembly line. Not exactly the American dream. The only joy I felt that I had in my life was partying hard on the weekends. The weekends were fun, but Monday mornings, not so much.

The company offered three weeks of paid vacation plus 10 days of paid sick leave, and believe me, I took every day, every year. Last year, in addition to my sick leave and vacation, I was out of work for four months after I stepped on a parts wrapper on a Monday morning and tore the ligaments in my knee. I went to my family doctor, and he said I had sprained it and put me in physical therapy three days a week. My knee hurt a lot but the pain pills my doctor gave me helped. The doctor told me not to drink while I was on the pain pills, but sitting at home all the time was pretty boring, so I'd invite some friends over a few nights a week and party at home. The booze actually made the knee pain better so I could walk a lot more, and the pain pills helped with the next morning.

After a month, I wasn't any better, so my family doctor referred me to an orthopedic surgeon who sent me for an MRI and then told me I needed surgery. A week later I had the surgery. After that the nightmare continued. A week after the surgery, my leg was very swollen and really hurt bad, so I started taking way more pain pills than the doctors had given me. I had prescriptions from the surgeon and one from my family doctor. Also, I found a couple of drinks with the pills helped a lot. Finally, I went back to the surgeon, and he said I had an infection in my knee and prescribed an antibiotic. I went through another week of hell and then went back to see the surgeon again. He put me back in the hospital immediately and said he might have to operate again if we could not control the infection. After five miserable days in the hospital, my mother who had been a nursing assistant called the hospital doctor and insisted he get an infectious disease doctor to see me.

The infectious disease doctor was very alarmed and said the infection had spread up my leg and if we couldn't control it, I might lose the leg. I need to tell you, that was not my best day. He started me on several IV antibiotics, and thank God, within a couple of days my leg started to feel better. They let me out of the hospital after two weeks and sent me back to physical therapy. After four months, I was back on the job, back to my life, and back to partying on the weekends.

After being at work only three months, I got called in to another meeting with the plant superintendant. He wasn't happy about my using more than my allotted sick days and vacation days and missing several Mondays since I'd been back at work. He recommended that I participate in the company wellness program. He said it as a recommendation, but I got the feeling that it was a bit more than that and that my job was on the line.

So, I filled out the online health questionnaire and got my measurements and blood taken. About two weeks later I met with a nurse. She told me I had high blood pressure, high cholesterol, and high triglycerides. She also thought I was depressed. She told me to go back to my family doctor.

My family doctor put me on two medicines for high blood pressure, one for high cholesterol, and one for depression. A total of four drugs. He also referred me to a counselor.

My counselor was great. She was also a single mom and sympathized with my situation. I continued to see her twice a week for a year. I would have kept seeing her, but after missing another three Mondays, I got fired. I couldn't afford the counseling because I lost my health insurance.

I was on unemployment for almost eight months before I found a job. Well, truthfully, I didn't really look that hard.

My new company had a wellness plan called 20/20 LifeStyles and if I participated, health insurance for my daughter and me was a lot cheaper. The wellness program at my last company was okay so I signed up. Looking back now, if I knew what I was getting into, I would have run away. But I am so glad I didn't.

It started out with the same type of questionnaire and blood tests, but then it all changed. I met with a doctor and a psychologist to go over my results which were the same as before because I had stopped taking my medicines since I couldn't afford them and didn't like the side effects.

The doctor strongly recommended that I enter a structured program, which was part of my company's wellness program, to deal with my blood pressure and cholesterol. He said he was pretty sure they could get it to normal WITHOUT THE PILLS! He said he would be seeing me throughout the program to check on my progress.

The program's psychologist wasn't as nice as my last counselor, but he was really smart. He seemed to know what I was thinking before I even thought it. He said he would be seeing me in this program. Well it took about two sessions with him before he remarked that I wasn't doing too well in the program because it seemed like I couldn't stop drinking. I told him I would stop, and he said we'd check on that next week.

A week later, I went in to see him all prepared to lie and tell him I quit but I could see by the look on his face when he asked the question that he knew the answer.

He talked about how my drinking had affected everything important in my life: my daughter, my parents, my friends, my job, and my health, and I started to cry. He was right! I had tried really hard to stop drinking for the program, but I couldn't do it, and it really scared me. He told me I had a serious problem with alcohol, but he also told me we could deal with that problem if I would do what he said. At that point I was finally willing to trust him and do what he said. He referred me to an out-patient alcohol treatment program, and I actually went. They told me I was a middle stage alcoholic. At 29 years old!

When I saw my psychologist a week later, I told him what the treatment center told me hoping he would say, "I don't think it's that bad." But, you guessed it, he said, "I know, I just thought you needed to hear it from both of us."

I finished the program as a superstar. I lost 25 pounds, my high cholesterol, high blood pressure, and depression were all gone, and I was completely off all alcohol and medications. During the 20/20 LifeStyles Program I met some new friends. My new addiction is exercise, and as a bonus my daughter has picked it up and goes on long bike rides with me on the weekends. She is just thrilled to have what she calls "real mom" now.

Well, that was three years ago and I'm 32 years old, my daughter is in high school, I've been promoted at work twice, and best of all I'm 3 years clean and sober. Life is good, and I am so grateful to my company and their wonderful 20/20 LifeStyles Wellness Program.

# THE ONE PERSON DISASTER

Cindy was much more than a problem employee; she was a problem that had wide-ranging effects on the company. Cindy clearly was not very good at her job, especially Mondays (when she was there). During these "bad days," she had the highest reject rate on the assembly line. But what about the "rejects" that she produced, which weren't caught by the inspectors. How many customer complaints and how much lost business did Cindy cause?

Because she was in withdrawal much of the time, Cindy wasn't much fun for the other employees to be around. She was very aggressive and verbally abusive to her co-workers. Additionally the other employees resented having to do extra work because Cindy didn't do it or was absent from work. Her supervisor had numerous requests from Cindy's co-workers for transfers, and several good employees left the company when they couldn't be placed in other units.

Add to this the inordinate amount of supervision and management time that was devoted to Cindy and to the problems caused by Cindy.

Cindy finally missed three Mondays in a row and that's when Cindy was finally terminated.

Over 7% of adults in this country abuse alcohol, 88,000 adults die from alcohol-related causes annually[55], and the cost of alcohol abuse is $224 billion annually. Another 9% abuse drugs (both illicit and prescribed).

55. *National Institute of Health, 2012.*

What this means is that 16% of your company's employees are potential Cindys. Even in a "drug free workplace" with adequate drug testing, drug problems still exist. Individuals abusing prescribed drugs with a valid prescription and individuals who know how to outsmart random drug tests[56] are still employed by your company.

## A BAD PROBLEM GETS WORSE

In 1988, the United States, recognizing the hazards of drug-affected employees in the workplace, passed the Drug-Free Workplace Act. However, with the legalization of medical and recreational marijuana, that problem has gotten a lot worse.

An average 150-pound adult, with a healthy liver, can metabolize an ounce of alcohol in one hour. That means that one hour after drinking the alcohol it will be completely out of their system. That is because alcohol is water-soluble and is easily filtered out by the body.

Marijuana's active ingredient, tetrahydrocannabinol (THC), is not water-soluble. Instead it is fat-soluble and is stored in the body's fat cells. The half-life of THC in the body is three to five days. That means after one use of marijuana, it takes three to five days to remove only half of the THC deposited in an individual's fat cells. Moreover individuals who use marijuana regularly can have THC stored in their system for up to six months.

This means that your employee who has a couple of glasses of wine with dinner is alcohol-free when he or she comes to work in the morning. However, this is not the case of the employee that uses marijuana on a workday evening or even on a weekend. They will be

---

56. *Almost all drug addicts know how to pass random urinalysis tests. These tests usually only "catch" occasional drug users.*

drug- affected when they are at work because the THC is still in their system and is slowly being released from their fat cells.

The impact of this fat cell storage of marijuana on your company's healthcare costs is far reaching. Most women stop using alcohol and/or cigarettes when they become pregnant. However, because marijuana stays in her body for months, stopping marijuana use when she becomes pregnant will not avoid problem pregnancies and damaged babies, which your company will pay for.

To make matters even worse (if that's possible), marijuana addiction is even more difficult to treat than alcoholism. Alcohol detoxification and withdrawal can take seven to ten days, whereas marijuana withdrawal can take up to six months. During that withdrawal the individuals are very angry, irritable, and demonstrate remarkably poor judgment, making it difficult for them and for anyone interacting with them.

# ALCOHOLISM AND DRUG ADDICTION

The 20/20 LifeStyles Wellness Program takes an integrated approach to dealing with alcoholism and drug addiction. Our first step is to educate the company's managers and supervisors in how to assess their employees for potential alcohol or drug problems. We teach them the key signs and symptoms that appear in a work setting. We also make sure all managers and supervisors can contact one of our professionals to discuss an employee issue that they suspect might be related to alcohol or drugs.

Next we educate employees using brown bag lunches, department meetings, pamphlets, posters, and online videos. We also make our professionals available to discuss any questions or issues employees might have. We have found that many employees actually come forward for help with their alcohol and drug abuse issues because of this process.

We also have chemical dependency treatment modules to treat alcohol and drug abusers.

Calculating the cost of alcoholism and drug addiction in your workplace is daunting. Alcohol and drug abusers are twice as likely to be injured on the job and five times as likely to file a workmen's compensation claim[57]. Treated alcoholics showed a 24% reduction in healthcare costs. More than 70 conditions requiring hospitalization (including cancer, heart disease, and AIDS) are associated with alcohol and drug abuse. And this doesn't begin to count presenteeism, absenteeism, effect on corporate morale, increased management time, and lost sales. The direct and indirect medical cost for alcohol and drug abusing employees is $20,000 per year.

Like Cindy, we have found that employees who have their alcohol and drug problems treated by their company's wellness program become their best and most loyal workers.

---

57. *Lewis, et. al., Center for Alcohol and Addiction Studies, Brown University.*

# 20/20 LIFESTYLES CHEMICAL DEPENDENCY MANAGEMENT MODULE

1. *Out-patient appropriate chemical dependency management program:*

   a. Intervention preparation and intervention with employer representative and/or family members plus chemically dependent individual.

   b. One year intensive out-patient treatment program.*

   c. Twelve visits with psychologist.

   d. Chemical dependency costs the company: $20,000/year.

   e. Program cost $5,200.

   f. ROI break even: 3 months.

   > * Initial 12 weeks: Three two-hour group sessions per week. Balance of year: One two-hour weekly group session. Entire year: One individual session per week. Treatment provided by Chemical Dependency Treatment Center.

2. *In-patient appropriate chemical dependency management program:*

   a. Intervention preparation and intervention with employer representative and/or family members plus chemically dependent individual.

   b. Four week in-patient treatment program with one year of follow-up group.*

   c. Twenty-four visits with psychologist.

   d. Chemical dependency costs the company: $20,000/year.

   e. Program cost $17,440.

   f. ROI break even: 10.5 months.

   > * Treatment provided by Chemical Dependency Treatment Center.

Does your wellness program have ANYTHING like this? If not, that might be one reason it's not working. The next chapter is a real life example of a company we recently helped: and yes, they actually LOWERED their medical costs.

# CHAPTER 13

## A REAL-LIFE CASE STUDY

## THE "ACME" COMPANY

This is a real life case study of the efficacy of the 20/20 LifeStyles Wellness Program. It is documented by Wells Fargo Insurance division, which was the insurance services provider to this company.

We will call this company "The ACME Company" (not its real name). ACME employs 391 full-time individuals and also insures 124 family members (a total of 515 insured). ACME is self-insured, and that self-insurance is administered by Wells Fargo Insurance.

Previously, ACME did not have a wellness program; however, they actively promoted wellness through their HR department. However, at the beginning of 2014, ACME implemented some elements of the 20/20 LifeStyles Wellness Program. The goal of this program was to cure employees (no families at this point) of their metabolic disorders.

ACME first presented the program to their managers, carefully explaining the 20/20 LifeStyles Wellness Program metabolic disorder modules. Then at regularly scheduled department meetings they explained the Health and Lifestyles questionnaire and the biometric screening to all ACME's full-time employees. They also explained that if employees participated in this program they would save on the employee portion of the health insurance premium for the year ($1,350). If the questionnaire or biometrics indicated they needed to participate in a wellness module, they would have to comply with that to receive the savings. These modules were provided at no cost to the employee. The result was that 86% of employees with metabolic disorders participated in and completed the appropriate 20/20 LifeStyles Program treatment module.

At the beginning of 2015, Wells Fargo was asked to prepare a report comparing ACME's healthcare expenses for 2013 and 2014.

*Wells Fargo told ACME that in 2014 the average healthcare cost per employee for companies in their local area rose 6.8% to $10,887*[58] *(not counting the cost of wellness programs). They also reported that ACME's annual healthcare cost per employee in 2013 was $5,880, but in 2014 it declined by 10% to $5,292 per insured. ACME had actually reduced their medical costs while other companies saw their costs continue to rise. The result was that ACME's healthcare costs were only 48.6% of the average in their local area.*

Although presenteeism, absenteeism, disability, and worker's compensation account for 76% of total healthcare costs, they are difficult to measure. Using the 76% guideline, however, ACME estimates its savings on indirect medical costs were $1,862 per employee in 2014 versus 2013. ACME also administers a job satisfaction survey annually and found that overall job satisfaction improved by 18% in 2014.

In 2014 ACME saved:

- Direct healthcare costs    $588 per employee
- Indirect healthcare costs    $1,862 per employee
- **TOTAL SAVINGS**    **$2,450 per employee**

Because ACME saved $2,450 per employee on healthcare expenses for 2014, they have not had to raise employee insurance premium costs, deductibles, or insurance co-pays for 2015.

Based on their outstanding success in reducing healthcare costs, ACME has committed to implementing all of the 20/20 LifeStyles

---

58. *Based on an average of 720 corporations.*

Wellness Program modules in 2015. That means for 2015 they will add the following program elements:

- Preventive talks at department meetings and brown bag lunches
- Incentive points for
  - Health and lifestyle questionnaire and biometrics
  - Vaccinations
  - Viewing educational videos and passing a short quiz
  - Attending educational talks
  - Reaching pre-specified goals on 20/20 LifeStyles modules
  - Maintaining goals previously reached for each year maintained (i.e., smoking cessation, weight loss, etc.)

ACME believes the use of motivational incentive points, redeemable for gift cards, will further increase employee participation in the 20/20 LifeStyles Wellness Program. The company also believes the incentives will motivate their employees to get all their vaccinations up-to-date.

Based on ACME's 2014 results, we are anticipating even greater healthcare savings in 2015. In fact, we are anticipating that ACME's healthcare costs will drop to under $5000 dollars per employee per year, a figure most employers haven't seen for a decade.

In Chapter One we told you how every attempt to control healthcare costs has failed. In Chapter Two we showed you how direct medical costs were only a small part of the problem, and in Chapter Three we showed you why traditional wellness programs are a waste of money. We have continually stressed that a "wellness program that works" must be staffed with competent professionals in many fields. Although some might think the implementation of this type of wellness program would be overwhelming, 20/20 LifeStyles has been doing this successfully for over 20 years.

Like ACME, some companies prefer to implement the program in a step-wise manner; only a few modules at a time. We understand the reasons for this and are more than willing to suggest starting points.

Hopefully this book has given you the information you need to not only "control" but lower your company's healthcare costs. We want you to use this information to improve your bottom line and the health of your employees. It's a win-win process that you can start today!

# APPENDICES
## APPENDIX A

---

## MANDATORY PREVENTIVE CARE SERVICES

The ACA mandates that the following preventative health services must be paid in full by all health insurance plans, without co-pays or deductibles. Furthermore, currently the government is trying to mandate seven "sick days" for each employee, so they obtain their preventive health services!

### Preventive Health Services for Adults
**Free preventive services**

All Marketplace plans and many other plans must cover the following list of preventive services without charging you a co-payment or coinsurance. This is true even if you haven't met your yearly deductible.

| SERVICE | PRIVATE PHYSICIAN: (Established Patient) | PRIVATE PHYSICIAN: (New Patient) | HOSPITAL-OWNED PRACTICE |
|---|---|---|---|
| Abdominal Aortic Aneurysm *(one-time screening for men of specified ages who have ever smoked)* | Part of annual physical | $75-$100 | $250-$381 |
| Alcohol Misuse screening and counseling | $70-$96 | $120-$182 | $324-$375 |
| Aspirin use *(to prevent cardiovascular disease for men and women of certain ages)* | Over-the-Counter $4-$14 | Does Not Apply | Does Not Apply |
| Blood Pressure Screening *(for all adults)* | | $28-$37 | $184 |
| Cholesterol screening *(for adults of certain ages or at a higher risk)* | $135. 50 | $293.50-$310.50 | $450 |
| Colorectal Cancer screening (colonoscopy) *(for adults over 50)* | N/A | $963-$1382 | $2316-$3210 |
| Depression screening *(for adults)* | Part of annual physical | $135-$152 | $206-$230 |
| Diabetes (Type 2) screening *(for adults with high blood pressure)* | $108 | $266-$283 | $465 |
| Diet counseling *(for adults at higher risk for chronic disease)* | Part of annual physical | $32-$40 | $215-$280 |

| SERVICE | PRIVATE PHYSICIAN: (Established Patient) | PRIVATE PHYSICIAN: (New Patient) | HOSPITAL-OWNED PRACTICE |
|---|---|---|---|
| HIV screening *(for everyone ages 15 to 65 and other ages at increased risk)* | $500 | $658-$675 | $870 |
| Immunization vaccines *(Recommended ages, and populations vary)* | | | |
| -Hepatitis A | $114 | $272-$289 | $362 |
| -Hepatitis B | $268 | $426-$443 | $517 |
| -Herpes Zoster | $178 | $336-$353 | $404 |
| -Human Papilloma virus | $384 | $542-$559 | $880 |
| -Influenza (Flu Shot) | $71 | $229-$249 | $319 |
| -Measles, Mumps, Rubella | $134 | $292-$309 | $382 |
| -Meningococcal | $261 | $419-$436 | $668 |
| -Pneumococcal | $73 | $231-$248 | $320 |
| -Tetanus, Diphtheria, Pertussis | $39 | $197-$214 | $337 |
| -Varicella | $391 | $549-$566 | $639 |
| Obesity screening and counseling *(for all adults)* | $45 | $85-$112 | $325 |
| Sexually Transmitted Infected (STI) prevention counseling *(for adults at higher risk)* | Part of annual physical | $50-$91 | $195-$220 |
| Syphilis screening *(for adults at higher risk)* | $103 | $261-278 | $424 |
| Tobacco Use screening *(for adults and cessation interventions for tobacco users)* | $70-$96 | $120-$182 | $324-$375 |

## Preventive Health Services for Women

All Marketplace plans and many other plans must cover the following list of preventive services for women without charging you a co-payment or coinsurance. This is true even if you haven't met your yearly deductible.

| SERVICE: | PRIVATE PHYSICIAN: (Established Patient) | PRIVATE PHYSICIAN: (New Patient) | HOSPITAL-OWNED PRACTICE |
|---|---|---|---|
| Anemia screening *(on a routine basis for pregnant women)* | $200 | $358-$375 | $542 |
| Breast Cancer Genetic Test Counseling *(BRCA)* *(for women at higher risk for breast cancer)* | $3,697 | $3817-$3833 | $3817-$3833 |
| Breast Cancer Mammography screenings *(every 1 to 2 years for women over 40)* | $120 | $142-$215 | $331-$575 |
| Breast Cancer Chemoprevention counseling *(for women at higher risk)* | N/A | $76-$168 | $195 |
| Breastfeeding comprehensive support and counseling *(from trained providers and access to breastfeeding supplies for pregnant and nursing women)* | Part of annual physical | $92-$119 | $160-$195 |

| SERVICE: | PRIVATE PHYSICIAN: (Established Patient) | PRIVATE PHYSICIAN: (New Patient) | HOSPITAL-OWNED PRACTICE |
|---|---|---|---|
| Cervical Cancer screening *(for sexually active women-every 3 years)* | $34-$48 | $153-$167 | $436 |
| Chlamydia Infection screening *(for younger women and other women at higher risk)* | $314 | $472-$489 | $645 |
| Contraception *(FDA approved contraceptive methods, sterilization procedures, and patient education and counseling as prescribed by a health care provider for women with reproductive capacity (not including abortifacient drugs). This does not apply to health plans sponsored by certain exempt "religious employers.")* | $30-$75 | Implanon (In-office procedure) $924-$1,030 | Inpatient Hysterectomy $14,290-$25,640 *Includes Physician, Facility, Anesthesia* |
| Domestic and interpersonal violence screening and counseling *(for all women)* | Part of annual physical | $135-$152 | $206-$230 |
| Folic Acid Supplements *(for women who may become pregnant)* | Over-the-Counter $4-$10 | Does Not Apply | Does Not Apply |

| SERVICE: | PRIVATE PHYSICIAN: (Established Patient) | PRIVATE PHYSICIAN: (New Patient) | HOSPITAL-OWNED PRACTICE |
|---|---|---|---|
| Gestational diabetes screening (for women 24 to 28 weeks pregnant and those at high risk of developing gestational diabetes) | $66 | $151-$168 | $274 |
| Gonorrhea screening (for all women at higher risk) | $30 | $115-$132 | $459 |
| Hepatitis B screening (for all pregnant women at their first prenatal visit) | $49 | $134-$151 | $221 |
| HIV screening and counseling (for all sexually active women) | $500 | $658-$675 | $870 |
| Human Papillomavirus (HPV) DNA Test (every 3 years for women with normal cytology results who are 30 or older) | $53 | $138-$155 | $347 |
| Osteoporosis screening (for women over age 60 depending on risk factors) | $100-$110 | $138-$153 | $238 |
| Rh Incompatibility screening (for all pregnant women and follow up testing for women at higher risk) | $50 | $135-$152 | $406 |
| Sexually Transmitted Infections counseling (for sexually active women) | Part of annual physical | $50-$91 | $195-$220 |

| SERVICE: | PRIVATE PHYSICIAN: (Established Patient) | PRIVATE PHYSICIAN: (New Patient) | HOSPITAL-OWNED PRACTICE |
|---|---|---|---|
| Syphilis screening *(for all pregnant women or other women at increased risk)* | $103 | $261-$278 | $409 |
| Tobacco Use screening and interventions *(for all women, and expanded counseling for pregnant tobacco users)* | $70-$96 | $120-$182 | $324-$375 |
| Urinary tract or other infection screening *(for all women)* | $19 | $104-$121 | $268 |
| Well-women visits *(to get recommended services for women under 65)* | $30-$46 | $158-$200 | $445 |

## Preventive Health Services for Children

Most health plans must cover a set of preventive health services for children at no cost when delivered by an in-network provider. This includes Marketplace and Medicaid coverage.

| SERVICE: | PRIVATE PHYSICIAN: (Established Patient) | PRIVATE PHYSICIAN: (New Patient) | HOSPITAL-OWNED PRACTICE |
|---|---|---|---|
| Alcohol and Drug Use assessments *(for adolescents)* | $195 | $280-$297 | $490 |
| Autism screening *(for children at 18 and 24 months)* | Part of annual physical | $221-$315 | $622 |

| SERVICE: | PRIVATE PHYSICIAN: (Established Patient) | PRIVATE PHYSICIAN: (New Patient) | HOSPITAL-OWNED PRACTICE |
|---|---|---|---|
| Behavioral assessments for children at the following ages:<br>-0 to 11 months<br>-1 to 4 years<br>-5 to 10 years<br>-11 to 14 years<br>-15 to 17 years | Part of annual physical | $127-$158 | $240 |
| Blood Pressure screening for children at the following ages:<br>-0 to 11 months<br>-1 to 4 years<br>-5 to 10 years<br>-11 to 14 years<br>-15 to 17 years | Part of annual physical | $28-$37 | $184 |
| Cervical Dysplasia screening<br>*(for sexually active females)* | $34-$48 | $153-$167 | $436 |
| Depression screening<br>*(for adolescents)* | Part of annual physical | $135-$152 | $206-$230 |
| Developmental screening<br>*(for children under 3)* | Part of annual physical | $74-$124 | $187 |
| Dyslipidemia screening for children at higher risk of lipid disorders at the following ages:<br>-1 to 4 years<br>-5 to 10 years<br>-11 to 14 years<br>-15 to 17 years | $33<br>*There is not a significant variance in cost from one age group to another* | $118-$135<br>*There is not a significant variance in cost from one age group to another* | $222<br>*There is not a significant variance in cost from one age group to another* |

| SERVICE: | PRIVATE PHYSICIAN: (Established Patient) | PRIVATE PHYSICIAN: (New Patient) | HOSPITAL-OWNED PRACTICE |
|---|---|---|---|
| Fluoride Chemoprevention supplements *(for children without fluoride in their water source)* | Sodium Fluoride Tier 1, Generic $5-$28 | Does Not apply | Does Not apply |
| Gonorrhea prevention medications *(for eyes of all newborns)* | Does Not Apply | Does Not Apply | $65 |
| Hearing screening *(for all newborns)* | $85 | $107-$124 | $190-$300 |
| Height, Weight, and BMI measurements for children at the following ages: *-0 to 11 months* *-1 to 4 years* *-5 to 10 years* *-11 to 14 years* *-15 to 17 years* | Part of annual physical | $85-$117 *There is not a significant variance in cost from one age group to another* | $249 *There is not a significant variance in cost from one age group to another* |
| Hematocrit or Hemoglobin screening *(for children)* | $21 | $106-$138 | $290 |
| Hemoglobinopathies or sickle cell screening *(for newborns)* | $11 | $96-$113 | $260 |
| HIV screening *(for adolescents at higher risk)* | $500 | $658-$675 | $870 |
| Hypothyroidism screening *(for newborns)* | $25 | $110-$127 | $311 |

| SERVICE: | PRIVATE PHYSICIAN: (Established Patient) | PRIVATE PHYSICIAN: (New Patient) | HOSPITAL-OWNED PRACTICE |
|---|---|---|---|
| Immunization vaccines *(for children from birth to age 18--doses, recommended ages, and recommended populations vary:)* | | | |
|   -Diphtheria, Tetanus, Pertussis | $77 | $235-$252 | $325 |
|   -Haemophilus influenzae type b | $55 | $213-$230 | $303 |
|   -Hepatitis A | $69 | $227-$244 | $317 |
|   -Hepatitis B | $33 | $191-$208 | $529 |
|   -Human Papilloma virus | $307 | $465-$482 | $803 |
|   -Inactivated Polio virus | $67 | $225-$242 | $315 |
|   -Influenza (Flu Shot) | $45 | $203-$220 | $293 |
|   -Measles ($390 if it is live) | $131 | $289-$306 | $379 |
|   -Meningococcal | $137 | $295-$312 | $386 |
|   -Pneumococcal | $246 | $404-$421 | $494 |
|   -Rotavirus | $198 | $356-$373 | $446 |
|   -Varicella | $391 | $549-$566 | $639 |
| Iron supplements *(for children ages 6 to 12 months at risk for anemia)* | Over-the-Counter $5-$15 | Does Not Apply | Does Not Apply |
| Lead screening *(for children at risk of exposure)* | $18 | $103-$120 | $281 |
| Medical History throughout development: *-0 to 17 years* | Part of annual physical | $222 | $222 |

| SERVICE: | PRIVATE PHYSICIAN: (Established Patient) | PRIVATE PHYSICIAN: (New Patient) | HOSPITAL-OWNED PRACTICE |
|---|---|---|---|
| Obesity screening and counseling | Part of annual physical | $85-$112 | $325 |
| Oral Health risk assessment for young children ages: <br> -0 to 11 months <br> -1 to 4 years <br> -5 to 10 years | Part of annual physical | $265 <br> *There is not a significant variance in cost from one age group to another* | Does Not Apply; performed in a Dentist's office |
| Phenylketonuria (PKU) screening *(for this genetic disorder in newborns)* | $12 | $97-$114 | $199 |
| Sexually Transmitted Infection (STI) prevention and counseling *(for adolescents at higher risk)* | Part of annual physical | $50-$91 | $195-$220 |
| Tuberculin testing for children at higher risk of tuberculosis at the following ages: <br> -0 to 11 months <br> -1 to 4 years <br> -5 to 10 years <br> -11 to 14 years <br> -15 to 17 years | $21 <br> *There is not a significant variance in cost from one age group to another* | $106-$123 <br> *There is not a significant variance in cost from one age group to another* | $215 <br> *There is not a significant variance in cost from one age group to another* |
| Vision screening *(for all children)* | Part of annual physical | $78-$84 | $130 |

# APPENDICES
## APPENDIX B

---

## MANDATORY PREVENTIVE CARE SERVICES TOTAL COSTS

If an employee were to have all covered preventive tests performed, the average cost of these procedures to your company would be:

|  | PERFORMED AT PRIVATE DOCTOR'S OFFICE | PERFORMED AT HOSPITAL OWNED MEDICAL OFFICE |
|---|---|---|
| Men | $1,000 | $2,200 |
| Women | $2,500 | $4,750 |
| Children | $1,200 | $2,640 |

# APPENDICES
## APPENDIX C

---

## RECOMMENDED VACCINATION SCHEDULES

The 20/20 LifeStyles Wellness Program strongly recommends having employees and insured family members receive all appropriate vaccinations. Just having all insured individuals vaccinated will substantially reduce healthcare costs. The following table contains the adult immunization schedule recommended by the CDC:

| VACCINE | AGE 19-21 | AGE 22-26 | AGE 27-49 | AGE 50-59 | AGE 60-64 | AGE OVER 65 |
|---|---|---|---|---|---|---|
| Influenza | 1 dose annually | | | | | |
| TDAP | 1 dose every 10 years | | | | | |
| Varicella | 2 doses lifetime | | | | | |
| HPV Female | 3 doses under 26 | | | | | |
| HPV Male | 3 doses under 26 | | | | | |
| Zoster | | | | | 1 dose over 60*** | |
| MMR | 1-2 doses under 55 | | | 1 dose over 55 | | |
| PPSV23 | 1 dose under 65* | | | | | 1 dose |
| PCV13 | 1 dose under 65* | | | | | 1 dose |
| Meningo-coccal | 1 or more doses any age*** | | | | | |
| Hepatitis A | 2 doses any age*** | | | | | |
| Hepatitis B | 3 doses any age*** | | | | | |

*If smokes or has asthma.
**If autoimmune system compromised.
***If other risk factor such as medical, occupational, or lifestyle.